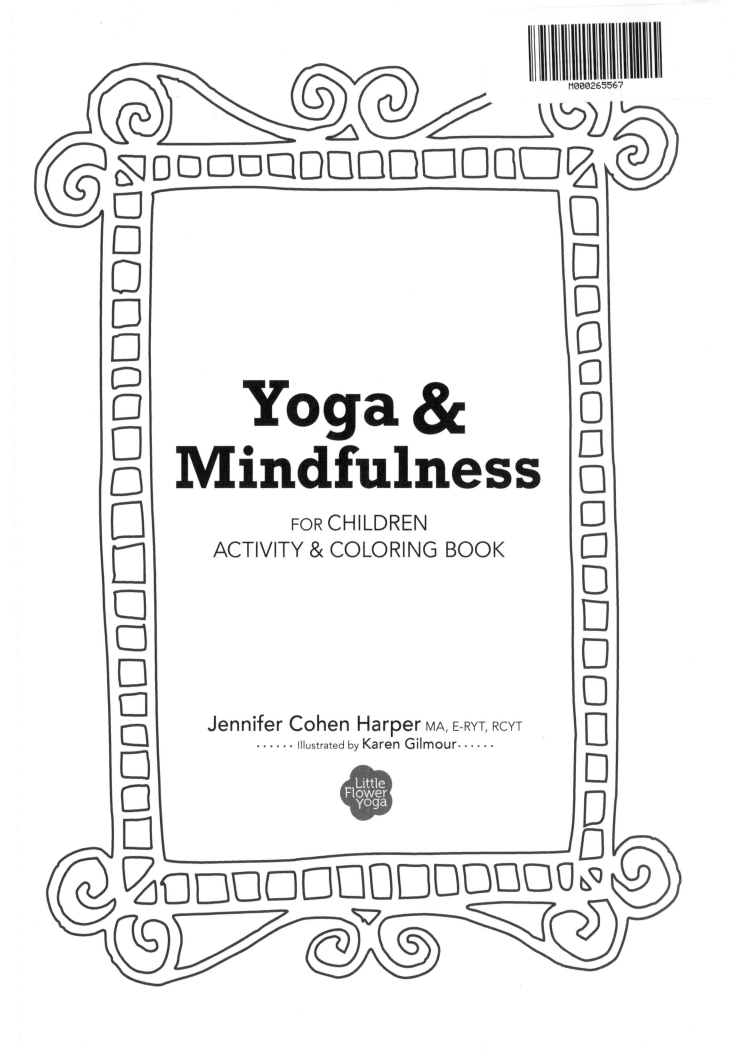

Yoga & Mindfulness

FOR CHILDREN
ACTIVITY & COLORING BOOK

Jennifer Cohen Harper MA, E-RYT, RCYT

· · · · · Illustrated by **Karen Gilmour** · · · · · ·

Little Flower Yoga

Copyright © 2017 by Jennifer Cohen Harper
Illustration Copyright © 2017 by Karen Gilmour

Published by:
PESI Publishing and Media
PESI, Inc.
3839 White Ave
Eau Claire, WI 54703

Printed in the United States of America
Illustrations: Karen Gilmour
Cover & Page Design: Amy Rubenzer
Edited by: Karsyn Morse & Jeanie Stanek

ISBN: 9781683730453

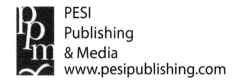

PESI
Publishing
& Media
www.pesipublishing.com

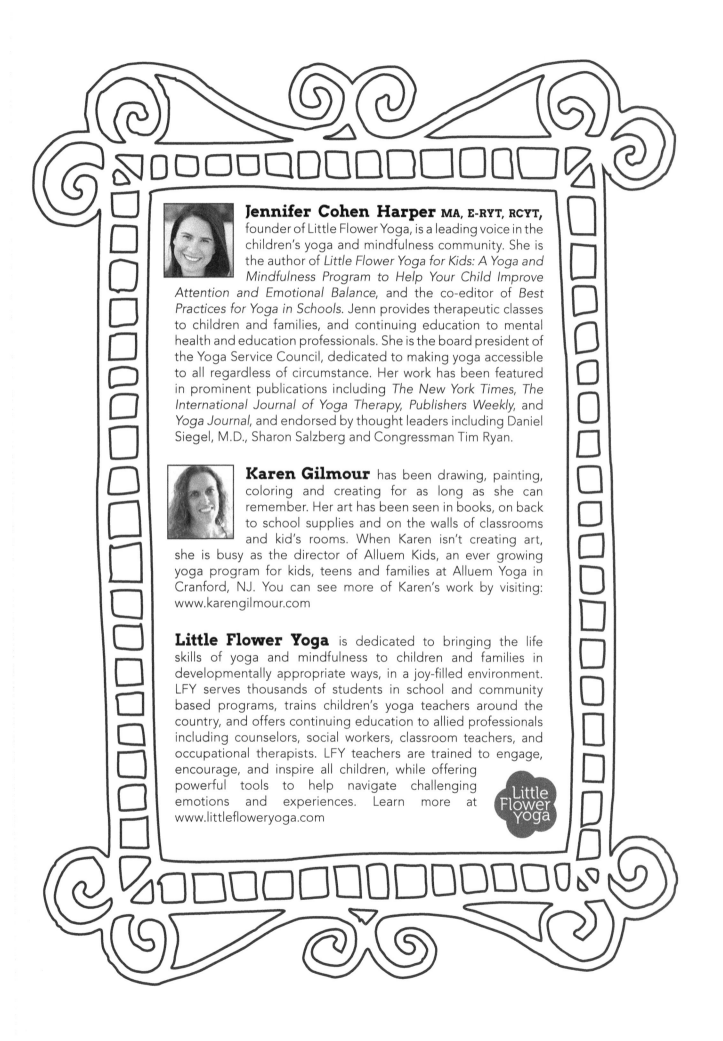

Jennifer Cohen Harper MA, E-RYT, RCYT, founder of Little Flower Yoga, is a leading voice in the children's yoga and mindfulness community. She is the author of *Little Flower Yoga for Kids: A Yoga and Mindfulness Program to Help Your Child Improve Attention and Emotional Balance*, and the co-editor of *Best Practices for Yoga in Schools*. Jenn provides therapeutic classes to children and families, and continuing education to mental health and education professionals. She is the board president of the Yoga Service Council, dedicated to making yoga accessible to all regardless of circumstance. Her work has been featured in prominent publications including *The New York Times*, *The International Journal of Yoga Therapy*, *Publishers Weekly*, and *Yoga Journal*, and endorsed by thought leaders including Daniel Siegel, M.D., Sharon Salzberg and Congressman Tim Ryan.

Karen Gilmour has been drawing, painting, coloring and creating for as long as she can remember. Her art has been seen in books, on back to school supplies and on the walls of classrooms and kid's rooms. When Karen isn't creating art, she is busy as the director of Alluem Kids, an ever growing yoga program for kids, teens and families at Alluem Yoga in Cranford, NJ. You can see more of Karen's work by visiting: www.karengilmour.com

Little Flower Yoga is dedicated to bringing the life skills of yoga and mindfulness to children and families in developmentally appropriate ways, in a joy-filled environment. LFY serves thousands of students in school and community based programs, trains children's yoga teachers around the country, and offers continuing education to allied professionals including counselors, social workers, classroom teachers, and occupational therapists. LFY teachers are trained to engage, encourage, and inspire all children, while offering powerful tools to help navigate challenging emotions and experiences. Learn more at www.littlefloweryoga.com

Little Flower Yoga

WELCOME

Welcome to the *Yoga and Mindfulness Practices for Children Coloring and Activity Book*. We hope you enjoy exploring it!

Yoga and mindfulness have a lot to offer to all of us. The practices and activities in these pages can help you get stronger and more flexible, manage feelings of anxiety, learn to navigate challenging situations without becoming overwhelmed, and much more. But perhaps the most important thing these practices can help with is the ability to be more connected to yourself — your body, your mind and your emotions. When you are more connected to your own experience, you can make better choices about how to care for yourself and how to respond to the world around you.

As you explore the activities on these pages, the most important thing is to notice what's happening with you. What are you feeling in your body, in your mind, and in your emotions as you try the practices? Does your experience change or stay the same as you hold poses, or as you try them multiple times? How does your body feel as you complete the activity sheets? Do you notice yourself always doing some types of activities and always avoiding others?

As you practice, do what feels right to you and trust your own body. If something doesn't feel right (if it hurts, makes you uncomfortable, freaks you out a bit) pause and check out your feelings, and then make a decision about what to do that works for you in the moment. Have fun, work hard, and be curious about your experience.

Jennifer Cohen Harper
Karen Gilmour

Little Flower Yoga

INTRODUCTION

The 5 Elements

The practices in this book are split into five activity types, or elements, that together offer you a complete experience of yoga and mindfulness. Explore the book however you would like, and if you want to try combining the activities on these pages into a longer practice, consider including one activity from each of these five elements.

Beginning Practices: You'll find a few pages with practices like Finding Your Yoga Seat, Mountain Pose, and Final Relaxation, that are a part of many other activities, and you might want to get familiar with them first.

CONNECT: Activities that help you connect to your own feelings and thoughts, to the world around you, and to other people

BREATHE: Different ways to use your breath, and explore the impact that it has on your energy level and emotions

MOVE: Practices that help you build strength, balance and flexibility, explore what your body is capable of, and develop your own personal power

FOCUS: Activities to help you notice what your mind is working on, strengthen your ability to focus and learn to manage distractions

RELAX: Opportunities for your mind and body to rest and restore

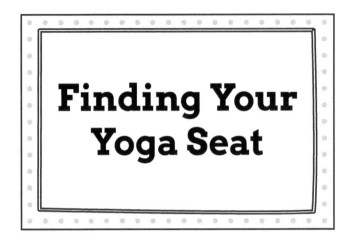

Finding Your Yoga Seat

Choosing your yoga seat is like finding a home base for your yoga practice. It's important that it's comfortable for you, and that you are able to rest in this position. You might choose a yoga seat for yourself that is on the ground or on a yoga mat, or you can have your yoga seat be in a chair. It's up to you, and may change from time to time. The idea is that you choose a way to sit that feels steady, and that lets you sit up tall.

Sit down and notice what your body is doing - Is it leaning to one side? Is it tilting forward or leaning backwards? Do you feel comfortable? Now experiment with different ways to place your legs and feet. You can try sitting with your legs crossed, or in a position called "Easy Pose" with one ankle in front of the other, or with one ankle on top of the other. If you are in a chair, try placing your feet flat on the ground.

Once you have chosen your leg position, sit up tall. Imagine what your body would feel like if you were very proud, and also a little bit relaxed. Each time you take your yoga seat, see if you can find this feeling.

Each time you practice, consider starting in your yoga seat with a few steady breaths.

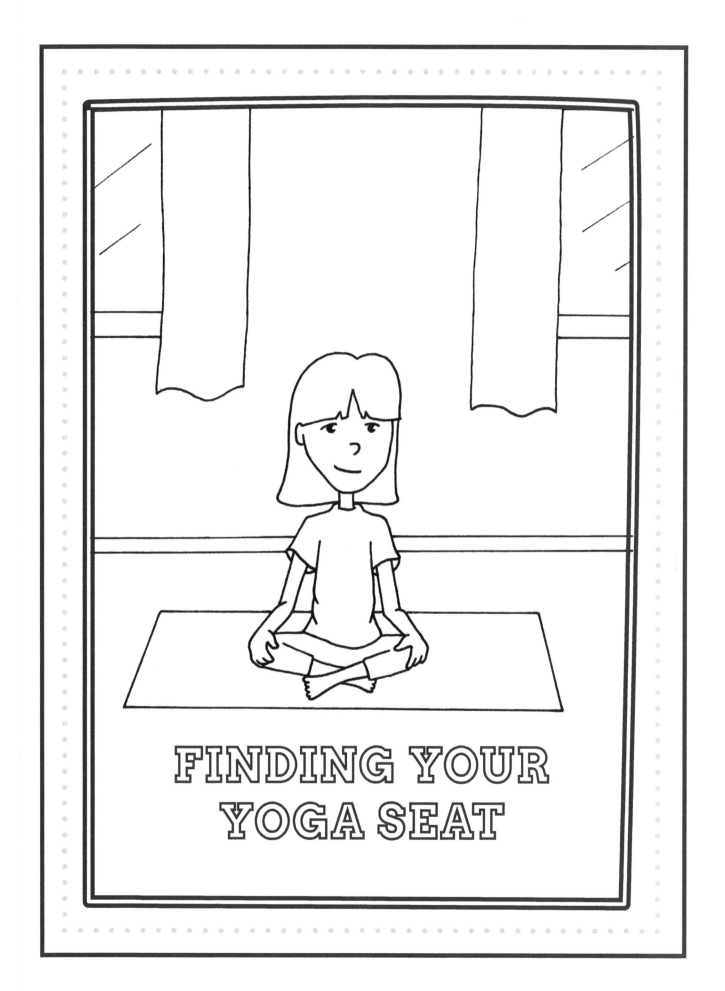

FINDING YOUR YOGA SEAT

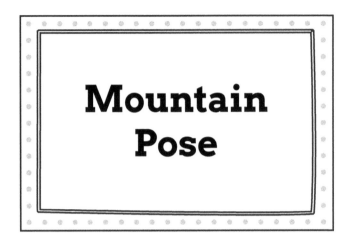

Mountain Pose

Stand tall with your feet just a little bit separated (about shoulder width apart) and your arms by your sides. Think about making your body strong and steady, but also a tiny bit relaxed, and definitely not stiff.

Wiggle your toes, then spread them out and place them back down. Imagine your feet feeling very heavy.

Check to make sure your knees aren't locked. Lift your heart so that you are standing tall, and then let your shoulders relax. Turn your palms to face forward. Let the muscles in your face relax.

Notice how you feel in this Mountain Pose. Every time you start a standing pose, consider spending a few moments in Mountain Pose first to get grounded and connect with your body.

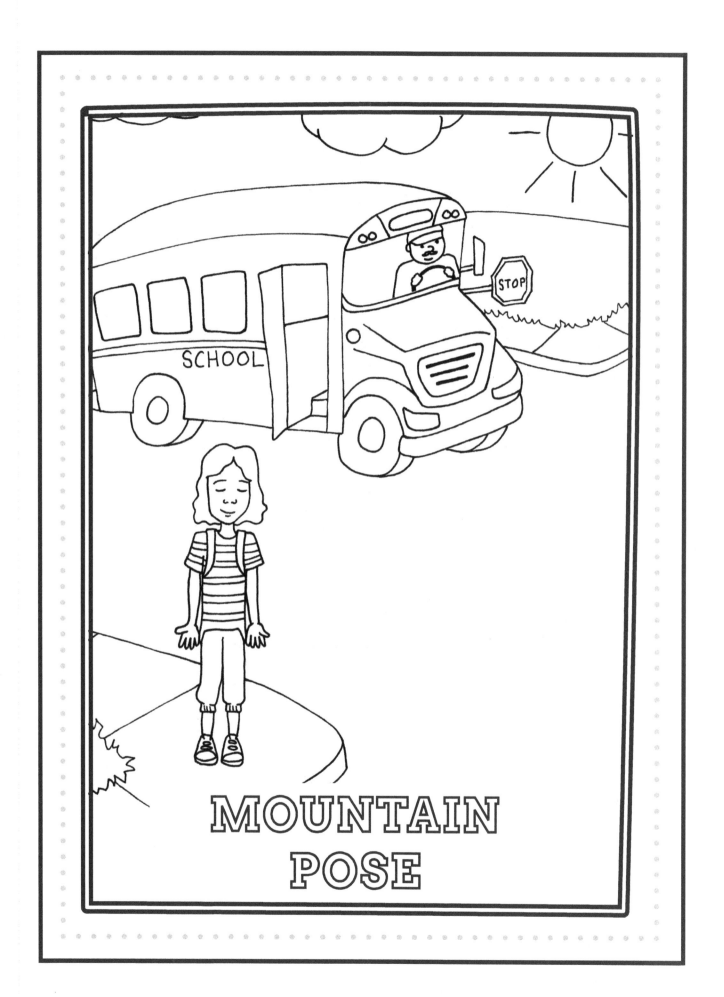

MOUNTAIN POSE

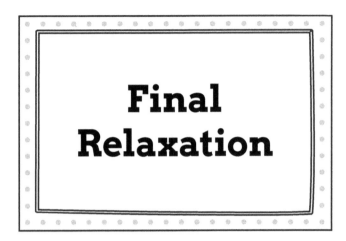

Final Relaxation

At the end of each practice session, whether you have done one activity or several, consider taking a few moments for a Final Relaxation. This means that you get as comfortable as you can, and don't do anything at all!

Try to keep your body still, and then just let your body and mind rest without any activity, visualization, music, or other distraction.

Final Relaxation is a time to just be. Sometimes this is challenging, as when the body gets still sometimes the mind starts to create a lot of thoughts, If this happens to you, just give yourself a gentle reminder that this is your time to rest. If it helps, you can focus on the sound of your breath. You can also consider putting a blanket over your body, and using an eye pillow if you have one.

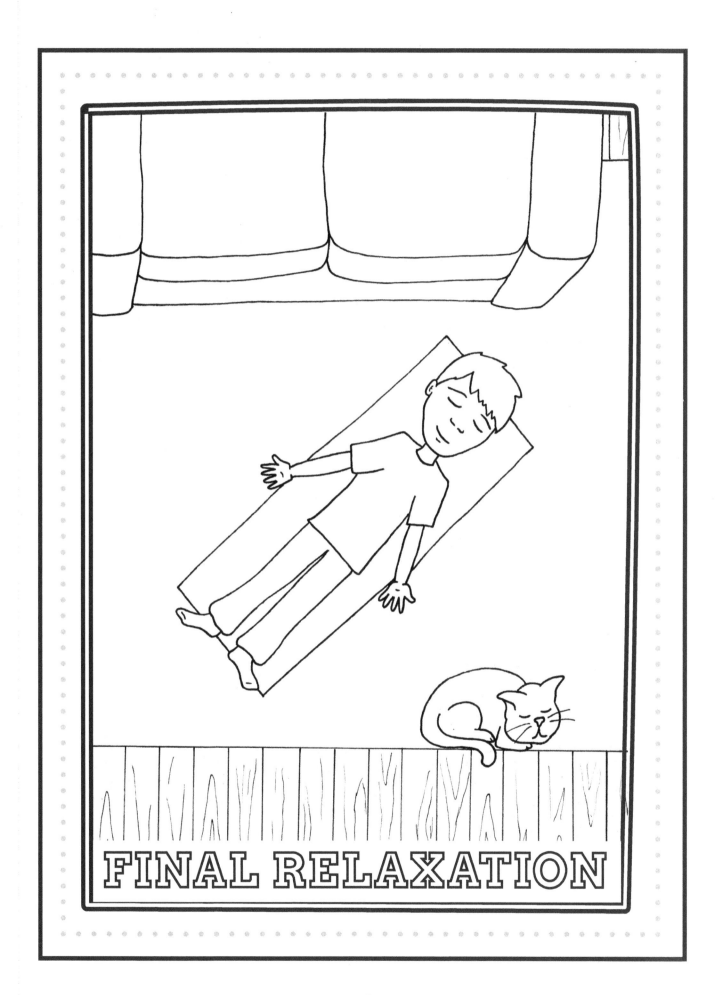

FINAL RELAXATION

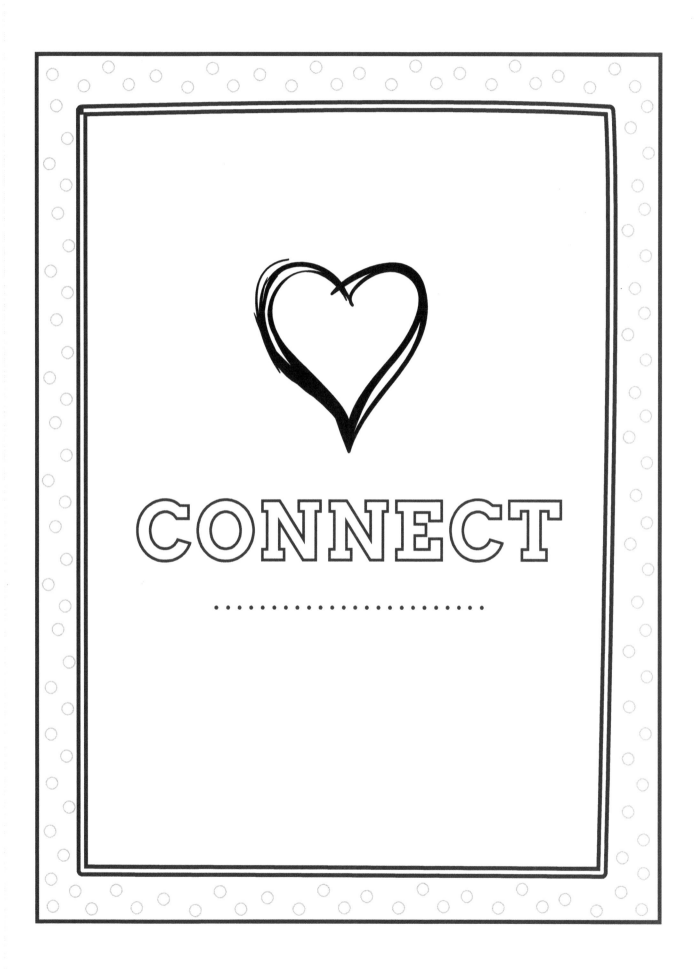

CONNECT

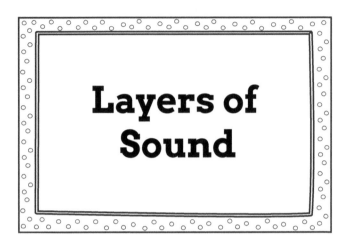

Layers of Sound

Find a still and comfortable position with your body. It's fine to sit in a chair or lean against the wall. The most important thing is that you are comfortable enough to be still. It may be helpful to close your eyes for this activity. If it doesn't feel right to close your eyes, let them rest on the ground in front of you or on one spot that isn't moving.

Take a slow breath or two to help you get ready for what is going to come next. The first thing that we are going to listen for are the sounds that are far away from us. Imagine opening your ears as wide as you can, and imagine stretching your hearing way out beyond the room you are sitting in. Listen carefully and find the farthest away sounds that you can hear. When you start hearing sounds, don't worry about identifying the sound or figuring out what is making the sound. Just notice it exactly as it is. Listen for as long as you like — 10 seconds is great to start.

Now that you have heard the farthest sounds you can find, bring your hearing in a little bit closer and find the sounds that are happening inside the building you're in.

Now bring your sense of hearing in a little closer to find the sounds that are happening just inside of the room.

Finally, bring your hearing as close as you can to listen for the sounds happening inside of your own body. After a few moments of listening to your own body, slowly open your eyes.

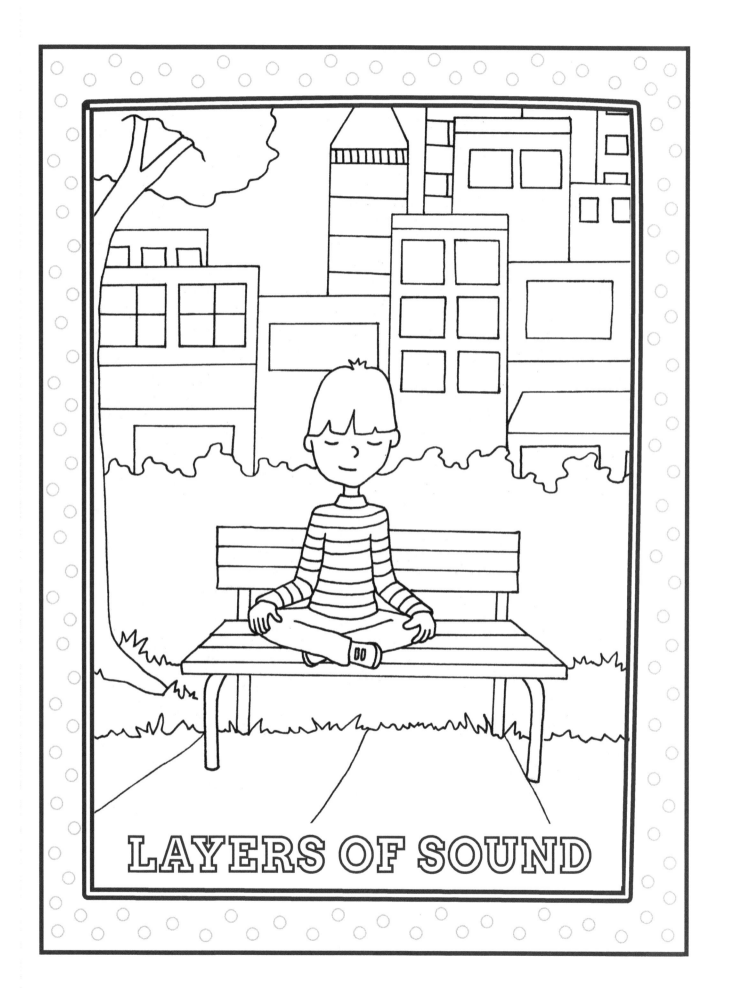

LAYERS OF SOUND

Layers of
Sound Exploration

What were the furthest away sounds you could find?
Use the space below to write about or draw what you heard.

What could you hear a little around you, or in the room you're in?
Write about or draw what you heard.

How did you feel during this activity?
What are some words that describe
your experience?

Can you imagine a time
when you might use this practice
at home or at school?

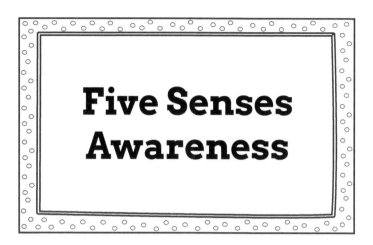

Five Senses Awareness

You can do this sitting or standing. First, bring your attention to anything around you that you can see. Look around. Take your time to notice what is in your environment….Now bring your eyes to rest on one steady spot, or if it's comfortable, close your eyes. See if you can remember what you saw around you. Picture it in your mind and hold it there for a moment or two.

Now imagine opening your ears wide and listen for any sounds around you that you can hear. They can be far away sounds outside of this room, close by sounds, or even the sounds being made by your own body.

Next pay attention to what you can smell. There might be good smells, or bad smells, or some of each in the air. Take a few slow inhales, and see if you can find one or more scents in the air around you.

Now focus on what you can taste. First notice what tastes you can perceive while your mouth is closed. Does the taste change if you move your tongue around your mouth? Does it change if you open your mouth?

Finally, bring your attention to what you can feel. What part of your body is connected with the ground? How do you feel the pressure on the place where you are being held? If you check in with the muscles of your body, can you notice any other feelings? How about the feeling of your clothes on your skin? The air on your face? Do you have glasses, jewelry, or anything else on your body that is creating a sensation?

Take a few slow breaths, and when you are ready, open your eyes or look up.

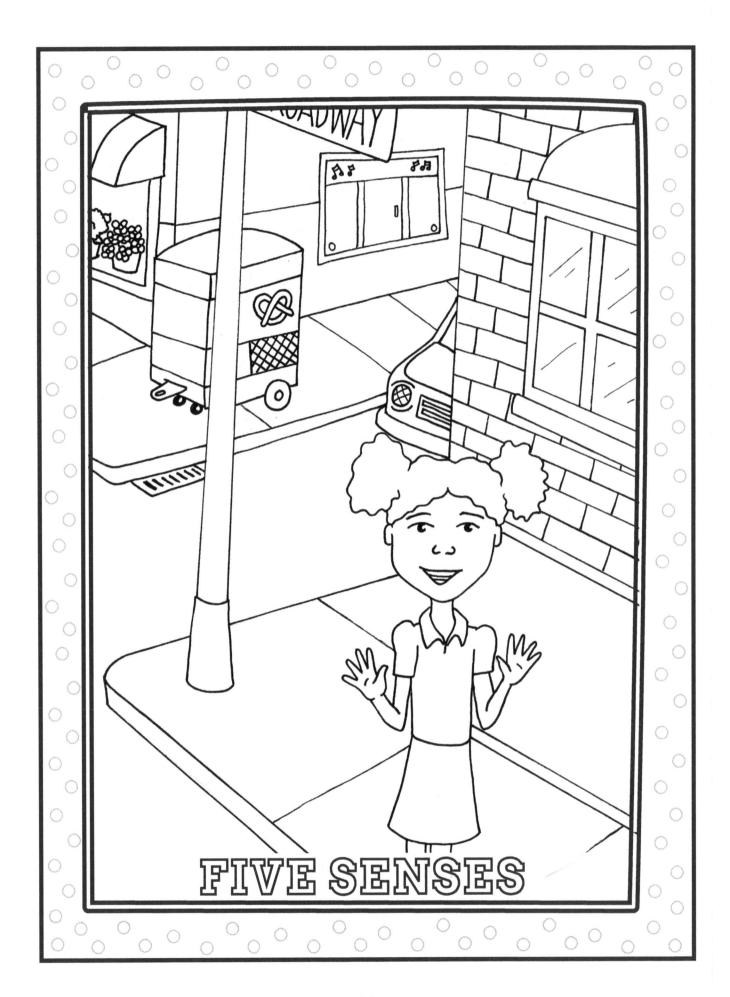

FIVE SENSES

Five Senses Awareness

Use the space below to write about or draw
what you can experience with each of your senses right now.

Seeing

Hearing

Smelling

Tasting

Feeling

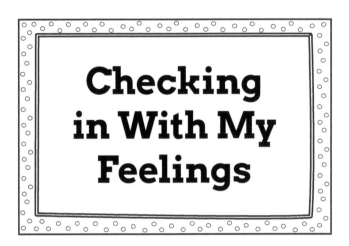

Checking in With My Feelings

Take a quiet moment for yourself to investigate how you are feeling.

You can sit or stand, but try to do so in a way that is steady and comfortable. Choose whether to put your hands in your lap, by your sides, or place a hand on your heart or your belly - whatever feels right to you. Focus on taking a few slow and steady breaths, and then ask yourself what emotions you're feeling right now.

You may notice that you are feeling more than one emotion, and this is perfectly normal. Sometimes you may feel two things at once, like lonely and angry, or embarrassed and frustrated. You may even feel two things that seem very different, like sad and happy or nervous and excited, at the same time! At other times it may be just one feeling that you notice showing up. Try not to worry about what is causing your feelings — it's enough right now to just notice them.

Once you notice how you are feeling, you may be able to notice that your body responds to your feelings. For example, sometimes we tighten our fists when we are angry, or our belly gets fluttery when we are nervous, or our eyes water when we are sad. Do you notice your body responding to your feelings today?

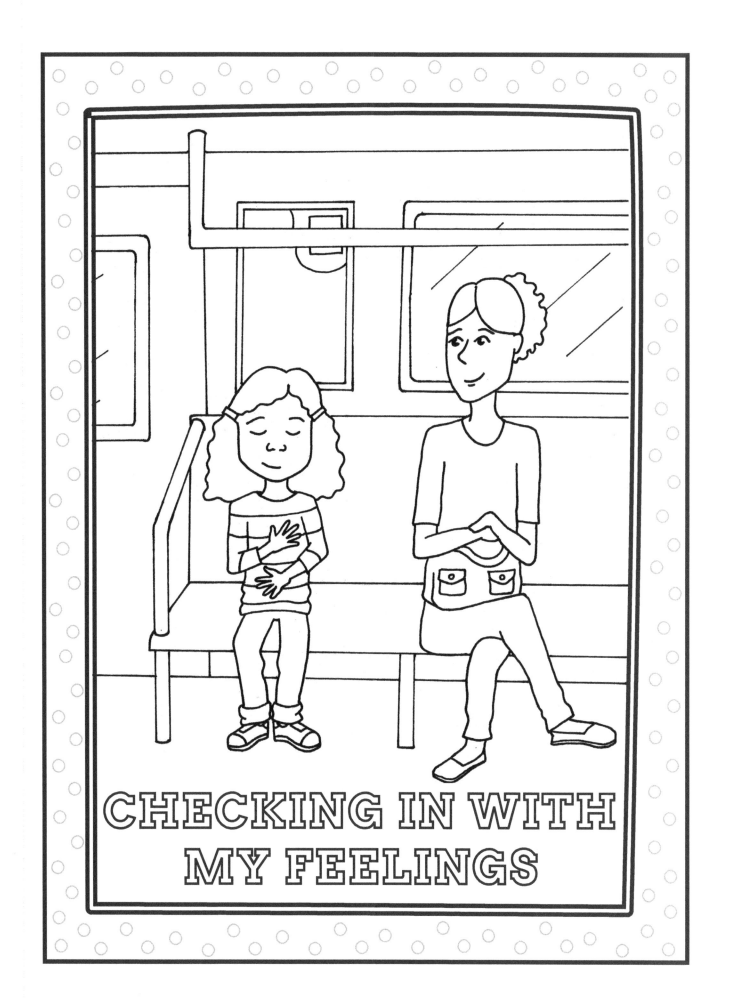

CHECKING IN WITH
MY FEELINGS

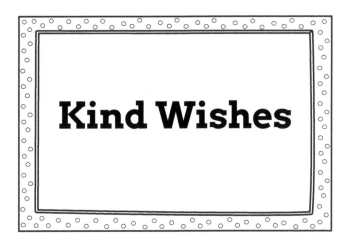

Kind Wishes

Sit up tall. Close your eyes or look at one spot that isn't moving. If there are other people in the room, imagine that you are sitting all by yourself. Notice what it feels like to sit with yourself.

Imagine someone that you care about very much walking into the room and sitting down right in front of you. What does it feel like to sit with this person?... Let's send them some kind wishes. Say to yourself, either out loud or in your mind:

….May you be happy...May you be healthy...May you be safe….May you be strong

How did you feel when you sent kind wishes to this person? Happy? Proud? Sad? Any other feelings? Was it easy or hard to send kind wishes to this person?

Now close your eyes again and imagine someone you think is a little annoying or frustrating. Maybe your sister or brother when they are driving you crazy, or a friend you had an argument with recently. It could even be a teacher or a parent. Imagine that person walking into the room and sitting down in front of you. What does it feel like to sit with this person?… Let's send them some kind wishes. Say to yourself, out loud or silently,

….May you be happy...May you be healthy...May you be safe…May you be strong

How did it feel to send this person kind wishes?

Now close your eyes, and imagine yourself sitting with a mirror in front of you. Look into the mirror and notice what it feels like to sit here with yourself... Now send some kind feelings to yourself, by saying ….

….May I be happy...May I be healthy...May I be safe…May I be strong

Notice what it feels like to send these kind wishes to yourself. Take a few steady breaths, and when you are ready, open your eyes.

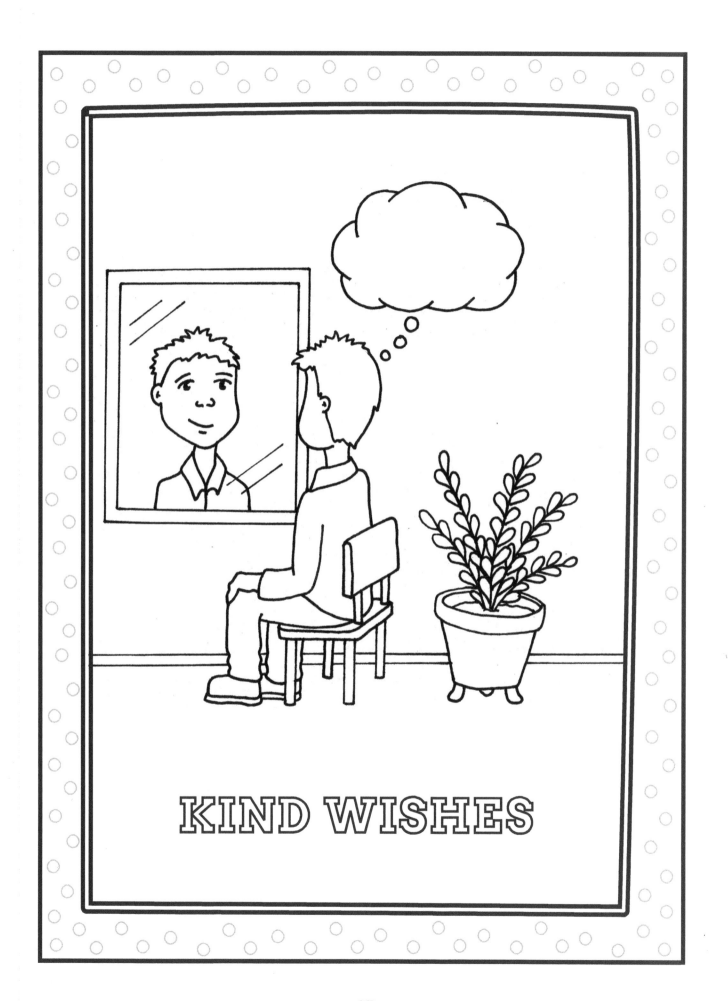

KIND WISHES

Kind Wishes Exploration

Who are the people in your life that it's easiest to be kind to?

Is it ever hard for you to be kind to other people? When?

Is it ever hard to be kind toward yourself? When?

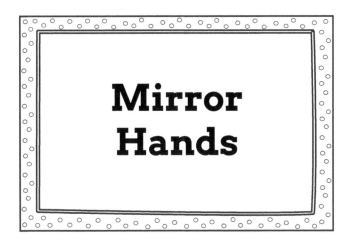

Mirror Hands

This is a partner activity, so find a friend or family member to practice with. Start seated facing your partner. Rub your hands together to bring some warmth to your palms, then bring your palms together with your partner's.

Look at your partner, but try not to talk. Begin leading your partner's hands — up, down, side to side — however you like. Your partner should "mirror" you and make the exact same movement. This activity works best if you move slowly.

After a few moments, switch who is the leader and who is the mirror.

Now that you have both had a turn in the lead, experiment with taking turns leading — but switch without talking! Can you stay connected enough to each other to "pass" the leadership back and forth. Maybe you are so connected you lose track of who is leading and who is following.

To add more of a challenge, you can slowly pull your hands apart (just an inch or so) and keep mirroring each other. Another option is to stand up and mirror each other's entire body.

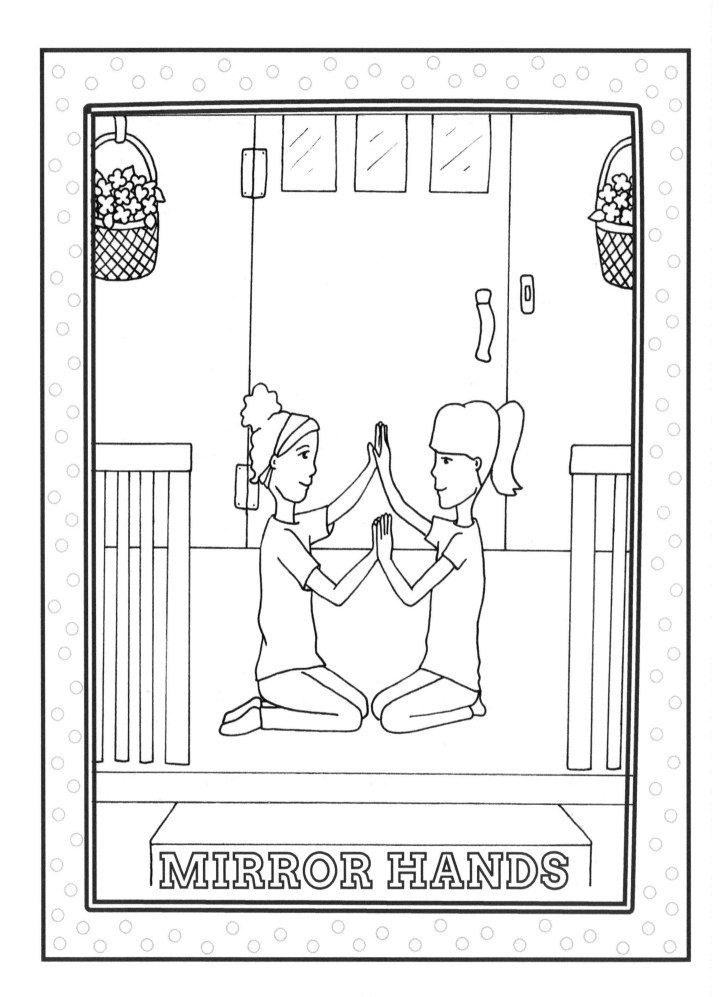

MIRROR HANDS

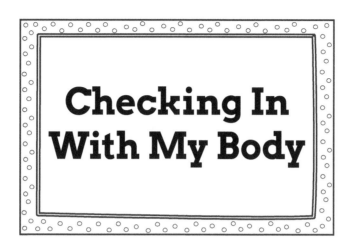

Checking In With My Body

It's great to practice this activity laying down if you can, but sitting up will work also. Settle into a comfortable position where you feel safe and supported. Take a few slow breaths, and turn your attention to your body.

Start with your feet and ask them how they are doing today. Notice if they feel relaxed or tense, comfortable or uncomfortable. Is there any pain or other strong sensations?

Next check in with your legs and see how they are feeling. Are the muscles in your legs working or resting? Are there any spots that feel tight or uncomfortable? Do they feel energized or tired?

Keep moving up your body to check in. How is your belly feeling? Full or hungry? Comfortable or uncomfortable? Is it relaxed or clenched? Can you feel yourself digesting food?

Now check in with your back and then your chest and shoulders. What do you feel? How much can you notice? How about your arms and hands? Your face?

As you check in with each part of your body, notice how it is doing, and consider whether the sensation has anything to tell you about your feelings. Maybe a flutter in your belly is a reminder that you are feeling nervous or excited. Or a tight and uncomfortable jaw might be letting you know that you are angry or feeling stress. If you're not sure don't worry, just check in with your body and notice whatever you can feel. Sometimes it can help to bring your hands onto the part of your body you are checking in with. After you've checked in, lay or sit quietly for two or three breaths.

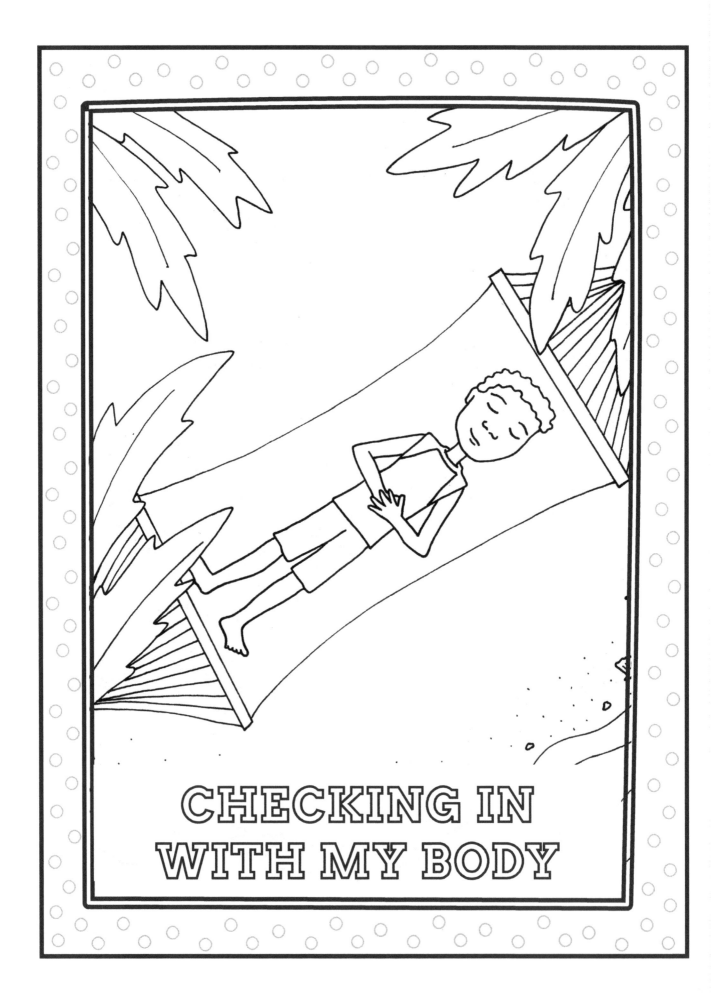

CHECKING IN
WITH MY BODY

Checking In With My Body

How is your body doing today? What can you feel?

Your Feet	Your Legs	Your Hips

Your Belly	Your Back	Your Chest

Your Shoulders	Your Arms	Your Face

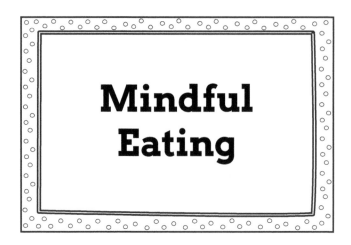

Mindful Eating

Every day we think about food, prepare food, buy food, and eat food. But sometimes we are so busy that we forget to taste our food! In this activity, we are going to explore all of the sensations of eating a piece of fruit. We'll talk about a strawberry, but you can try this with any food you'd like.

Pick up a strawberry. Don't worry—you are going to get to eat it but not just yet. First explore the strawberry with your hands. Notice how heavy or light it is. Feel the texture of the skin and notice its temperature.

After you explore your strawberry with your sense of touch, start to explore it with your sense of sight. Notice the color — is it even all the way around or does the color have variation in it? Notice if the skin is shiny or dull. Check out the seeds and the stem.

Now see if you can smell your strawberry. First just hold it up to your nose. Then try scratching the skin and notice if it smells any different. We have two senses left to explore with: hearing and tasting.

To listen, hold the berry up to your ear, and lightly scratch the surface. Can you hear any sounds?

Now it's time to use your sense of taste! Go ahead put the berry in your mouth, or if it's large take one bite. Try not to chew at first. Notice what the fruit feels like in your mouth, and what it tastes like on the outside. When you are ready to take a bite do it slowly and notice everything — the taste, the feeling, your thoughts (maybe you can hear more sounds?). Does the berry taste different on the inside and the outside? Can you feel it moving down your throat as you swallow?

When you are finished swallowing, start over with another bite, or another berry, and notice if there is any difference between the two.

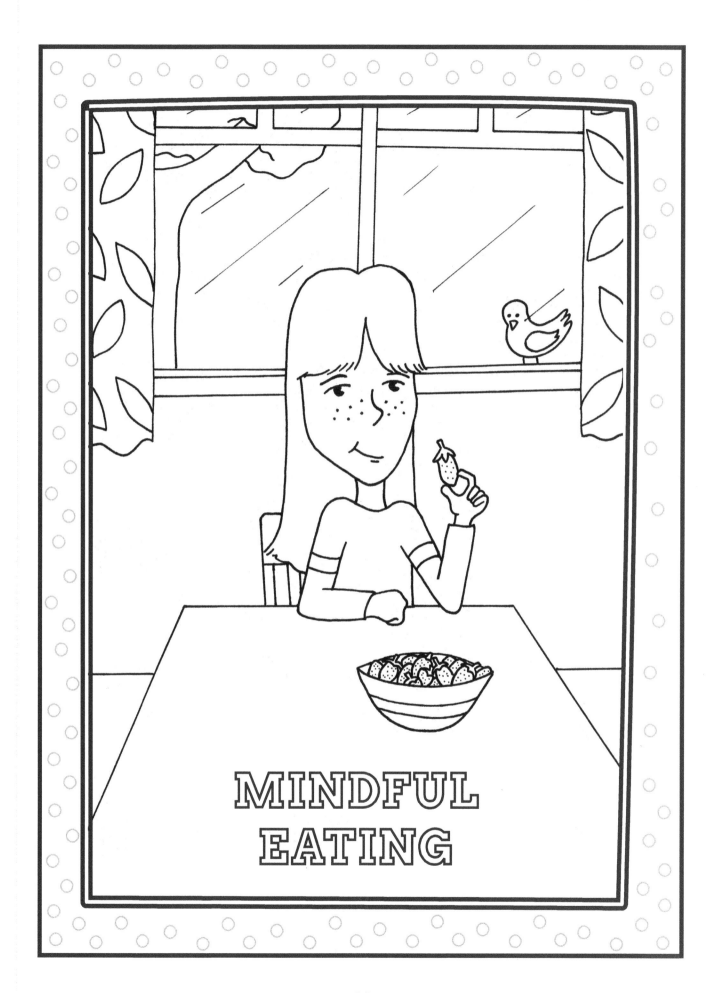

MINDFUL
EATING

Mindful Eating Exploration

What did you choose to eat? _____

How did it:

    Feel: _____

    _____

    _____

    Look: _____

    _____

    _____

    Smell: _____

    _____

    _____

    Sound: _____

    _____

    _____

    Taste: _____

    _____

    _____

Did you notice anything else? _____

_____

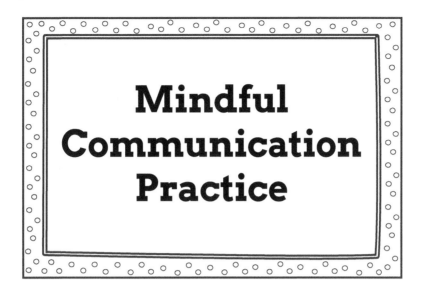

Mindful Communication Practice

Having another person listen carefully and compassionately to what you are saying, and listening to them in return, is an important part of connecting to each other. When you are an active listener for another person, you help them find their own words. Often when people talk to each other we are distracted, or thinking about what we are going to say in response to what we are hearing. In this activity you will work with a partner to practice listening, and experience talking while someone is listening to you.

Find a friend or family member to share this practice with. Choose one of the questions below to ask each other. Set a timer for a specific amount of time (about 3 minutes would be a good start) and take turns being the speaker and the listener for that set amount of time each. When you are listening, be an active listener and stay tuned in to your partner — you can nod, smile, say things like uh huh and I hear you. But don't ask questions, interrupt, or make comments about what is being said.

While you are the listener, pay attention to your partner but also notice your own thoughts, feelings and body while you are listening. Is listening challenging? Are you wanting to ask a question? Are you getting anxious for your turn? When you are the speaker, notice how it feels to talk without interruptions or questions. If there is some silence that is ok also, just wait until either the speaker wants to talk again, or the timer is finished.

Possible questions and topics for mindful communication:

- What are some things that make you happy or feel meaningful in your life?
- How do you manage when you are feeling upset or overwhelmed?
- What is something you are proud of?

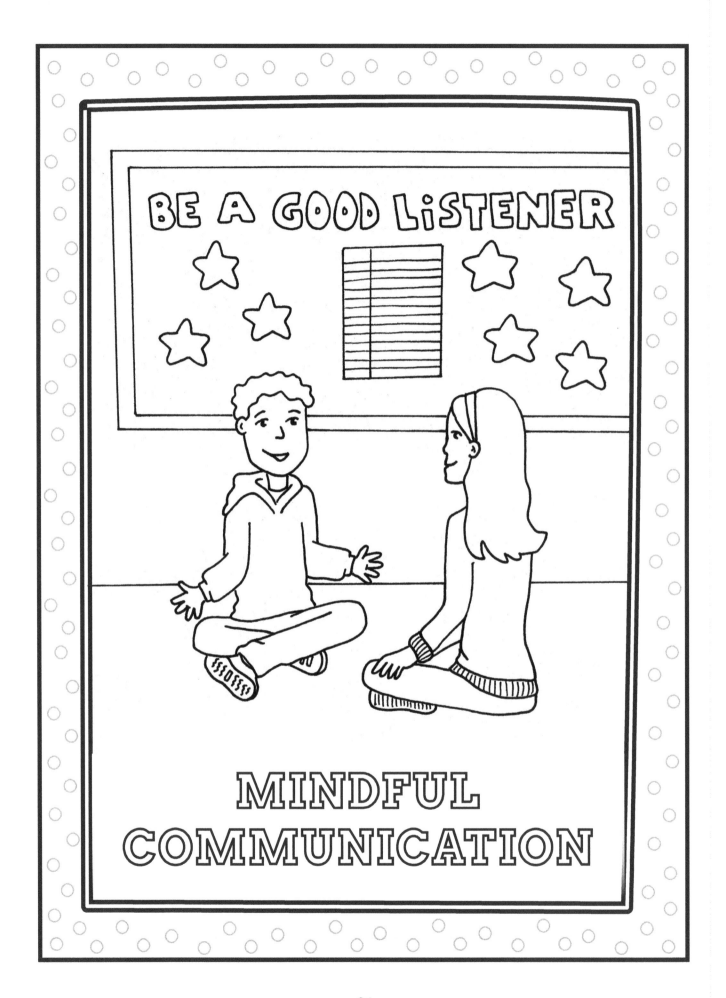

Mindful Communication Exploration

How did you feel when you were the listener? _____

    Your Body: _____

    _____

    Your Mind: _____

    _____

    Your Feelings: _____

    _____

. . . .

How did you feel when you were the speaker? _____

    Your Body: _____

    _____

    Your Mind: _____

    _____

    Your Feelings: _____

    _____

. . . .

Did you notice anything else? _____

_____

_____

_____

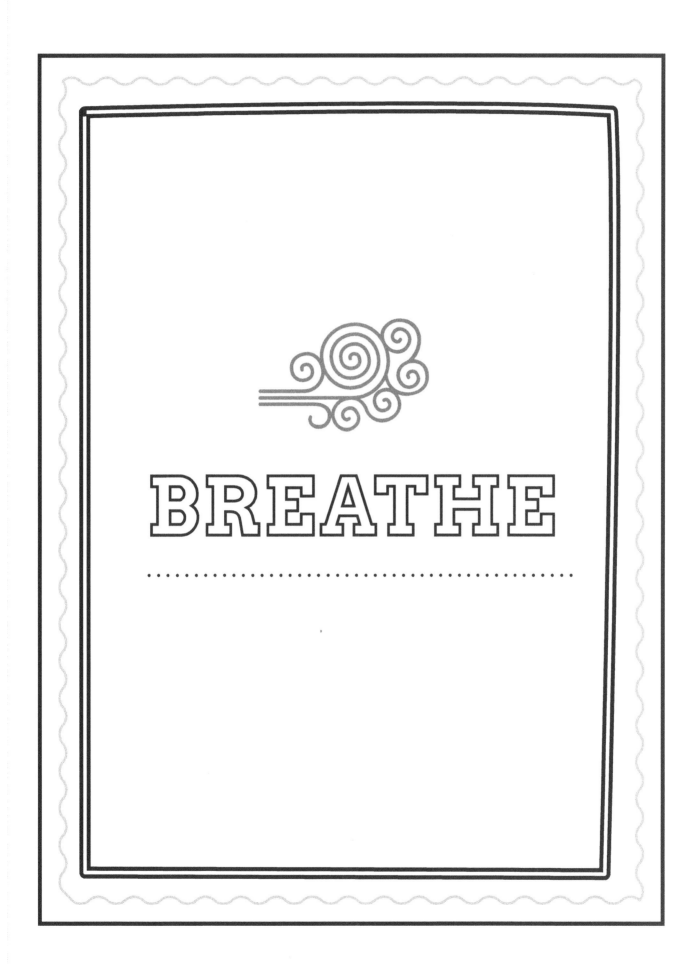

BREATHE

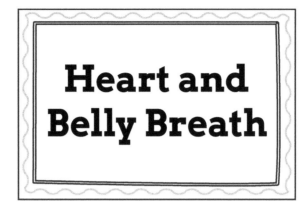

Heart and Belly Breath

Bring one hand to your belly and one hand to your heart. You can do this practice with your eyes open or closed, and your body sitting up or laying down.

Notice the feeling of your hands resting on your heart and belly. Let your hands be heavy on your body so that you can really feel the connection. Can you feel your breath moving in your body? Just pay attention to the sensation of your breathing, without trying to change it.

After a few moments, start to slow your breath down, and make your breath steady and even, so that your inhale and exhale are the same length. Breathe in and out through your nose. Can you feel your breath moving through your body? Notice any sensations, and, when you are ready, bring your hands down.

Calming Breath:

If you would like to help your body get even more settled, you can experiment with making your exhale longer than your inhale. This helps your body turn on something called the "relaxation response" and may help you to feel calmer.

Begin by silently counting your breathing pattern, for example inhale one, two; exhale one, two…. Make sure that the count isn't too long and that you can comfortably inhale and exhale. Once you are breathing at a steady pace for a few rounds, start to make your exhale longer then your inhale. You can start by counting inhale one, two; exhale one, two, three. If this feels okay, try inhale one, two; exhale one, two, three, four … Continue this pattern for as long as you feel comfortable. When you're ready to finish, come back to an even breath for a round or two, and then open your eyes or look up.

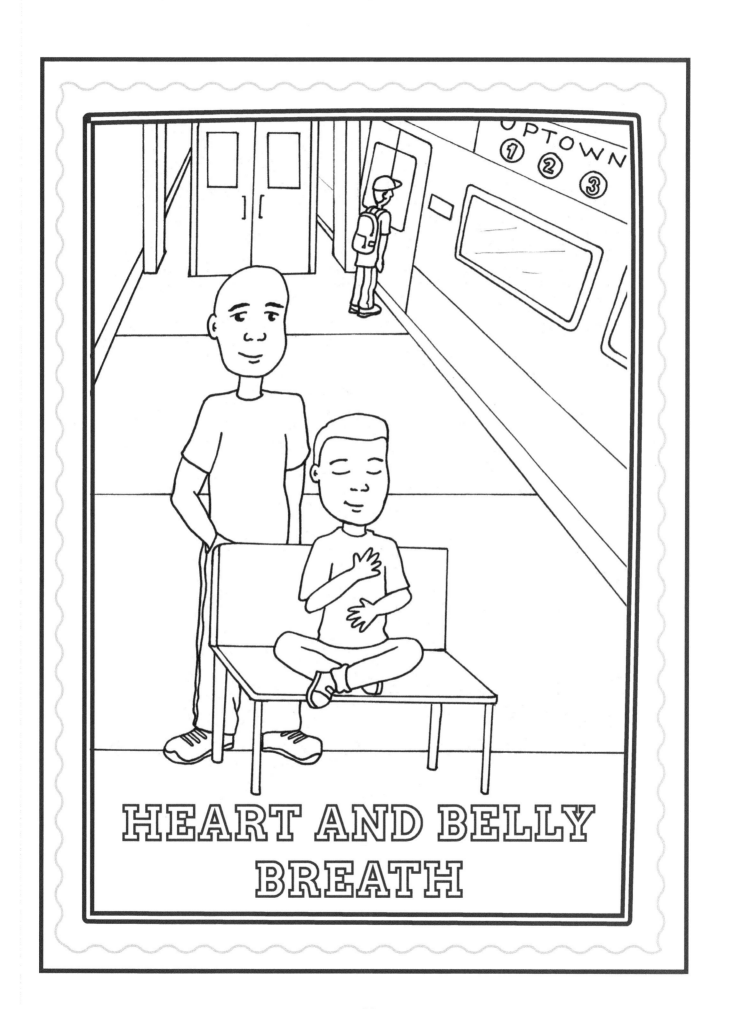

HEART AND BELLY BREATH

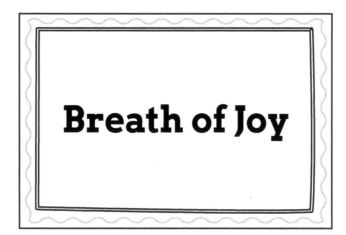

Breath of Joy

Start standing, with your feet hip-width apart and your knees gently bent. You are going to breathe in through your nose three times, using a short, quick inhale, and then out through your mouth with a gentle, longer "haaaaa" sound.

On your first inhale, bring your arms straight out in front of you. Then inhale again while bringing your arms out to the sides. Finally inhale again while swinging your arms straight overhead. When you're ready to exhale, let your arms swing down alongside your body, fold forward, and let out all of your air through your mouth. Try making a "haaaaa" sound as you empty all of your breath.

Repeat this pattern several times….inhale, inhale, inhale, haaaa.......Start off slowly, and when you get the rhythm of the breath you can go a little bit faster. When you're done, stand steady in Mountain Pose for a moment and take a slow steady breath or two as you notice the energy in your body.

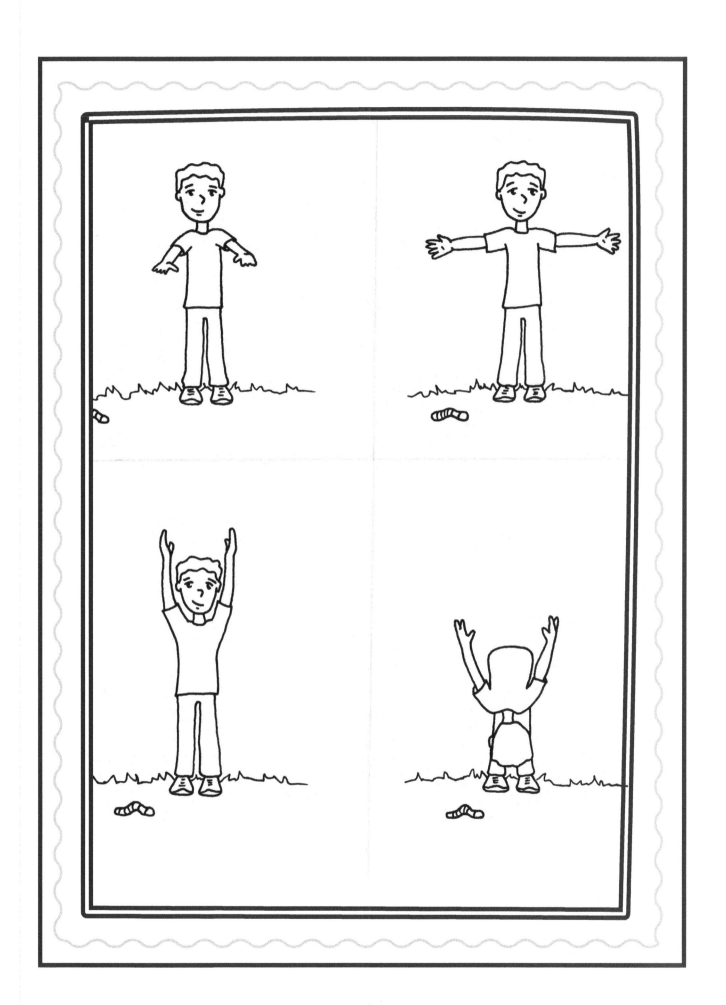

What Brings You Joy?

What are the things in your life that bring you the most joy?
Use the space below to write or draw.

People

Places

Things

Experiences

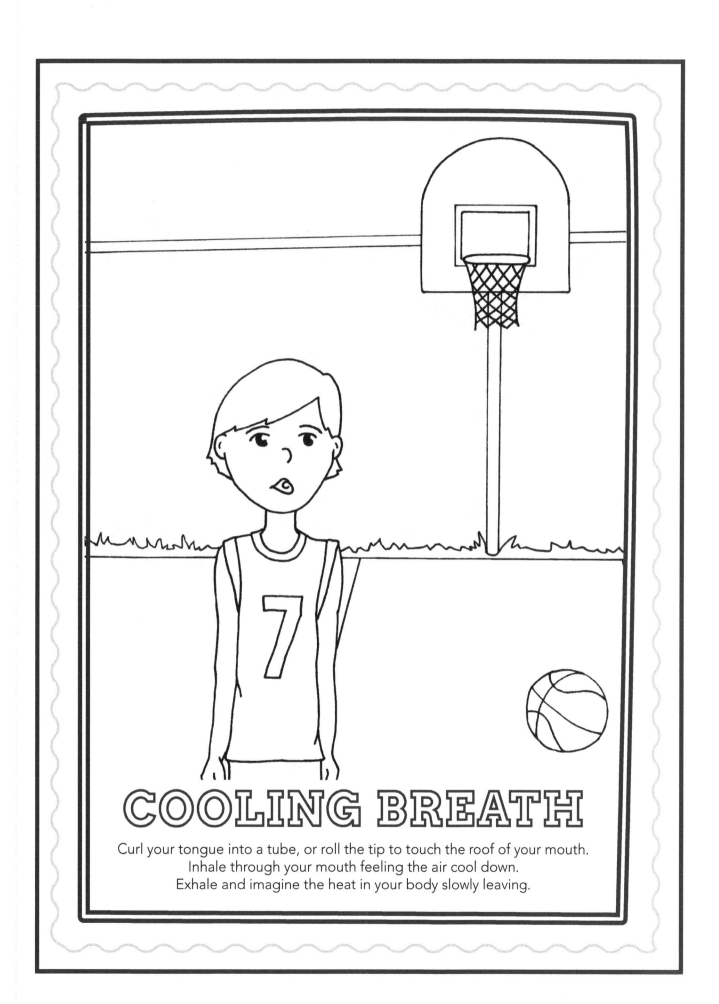

COOLING BREATH

Curl your tongue into a tube, or roll the tip to touch the roof of your mouth.
Inhale through your mouth feeling the air cool down.
Exhale and imagine the heat in your body slowly leaving.

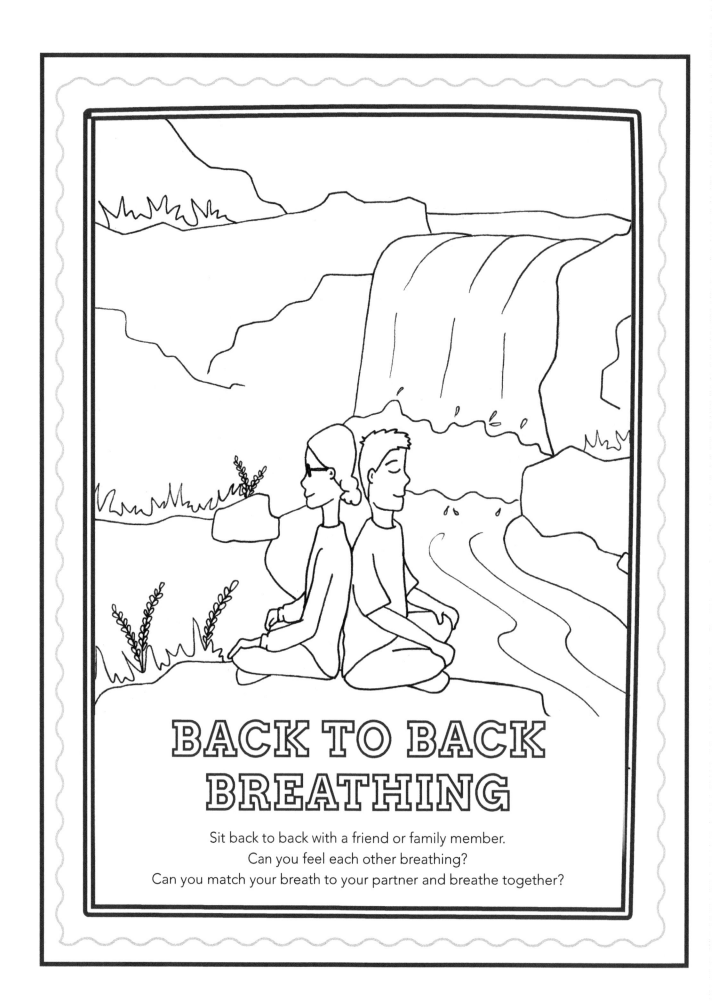

BACK TO BACK BREATHING

Sit back to back with a friend or family member.
Can you feel each other breathing?
Can you match your breath to your partner and breathe together?

Who Has Your Back?

We all need someone in our lives that has our back no matter what.
Who is that person for you? Draw or write about them in the space below.

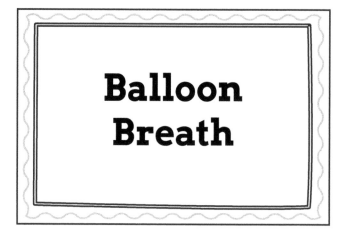

Balloon Breath

Sit on the floor or in a chair, with your back straight and tall. Place your hands on your knees and start to breathe in and out through your nose. Imagine that your body is a balloon, and with each breath in you are filling yourself completely with air.

As you breathe in, arch your back, let your chest and belly soften and move forward, and look up. This is a modified form of Cow Pose. As you breathe out, pull your belly button in, round your back, and look down toward your belly. This is a modified form of Cat Pose. Repeat this movement and breath pattern several times, breathing in to fill up your body and breathing out to deflate it.

On your next inhale, open your chest, but this time bring your arms up and over your head as well. Make your body very big and full. As you breathe out, bring your arms back down and as you round your back and pull in your belly, wrap your arms around yourself in a hug. Continue for a few rounds, breathing in to fill yourself up and get very big, and breathing out to make yourself as small as you can be. With each exhale, try alternating which arm is on top during your hug.

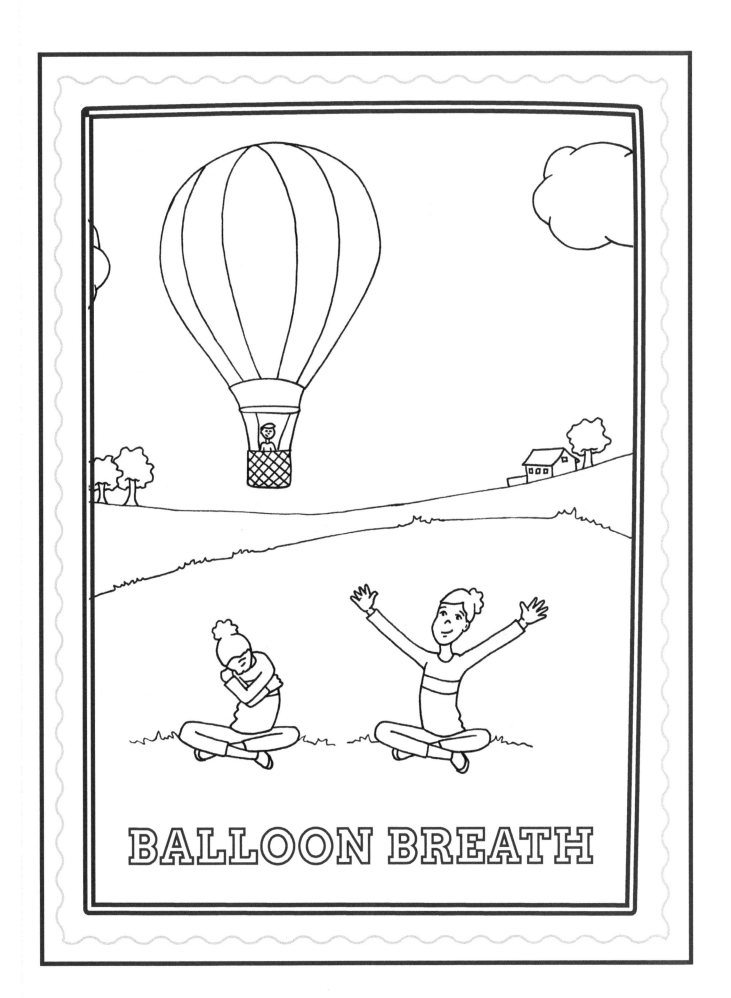

BALLOON BREATH

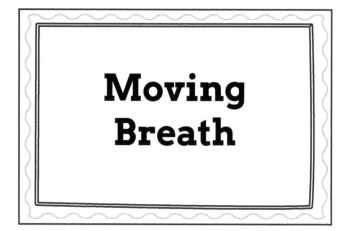

Moving Breath

Stand in Mountain Pose, strong and steady with your arms down by your sides. Take three slow breaths in and out through your nose. Notice how your body moves as you breathe. As you inhale let your body soften and your belly and chest expand, and as you exhale notice your chest fall.

Now as you inhale raise your arms overhead. Take the whole length of your breath to raise your arms. See if you can time it so that your arms are straight up just when you have finished your inhale. Then lower them down as you exhale. Repeat this coordination of your breath and your movement at least three times, move if you'd like.

If you want to try more breath to movement coordination, experiment with lifting your arms as you inhale, and folding forward over your legs as you exhale.

Finish the way you started, with three breaths in Mountain Pose.

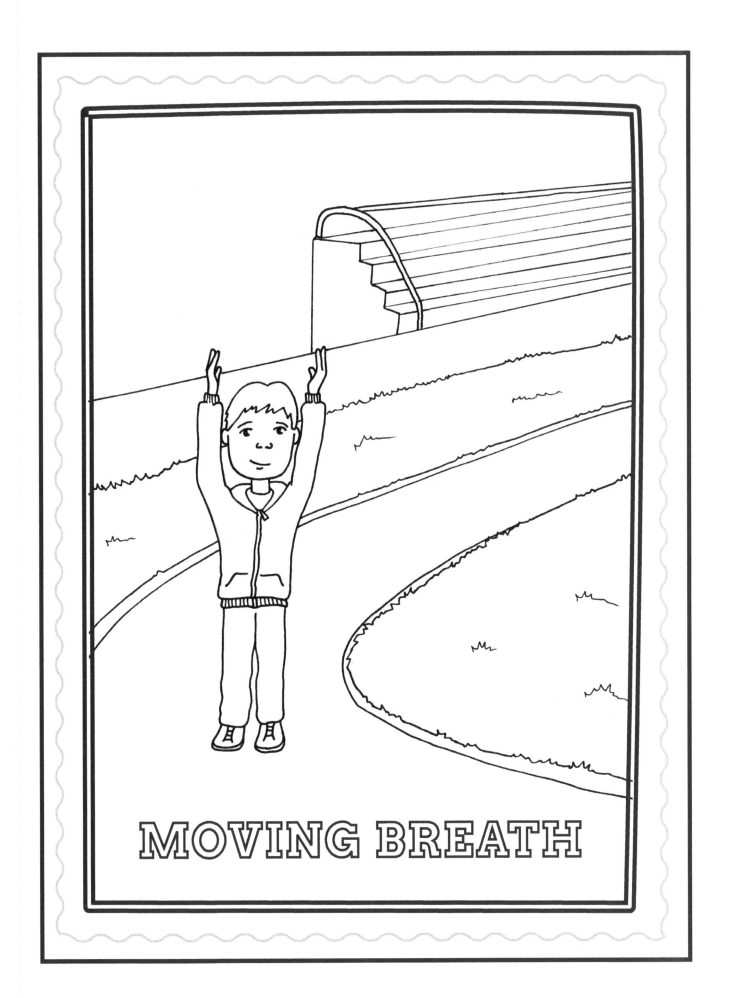

MOVING BREATH

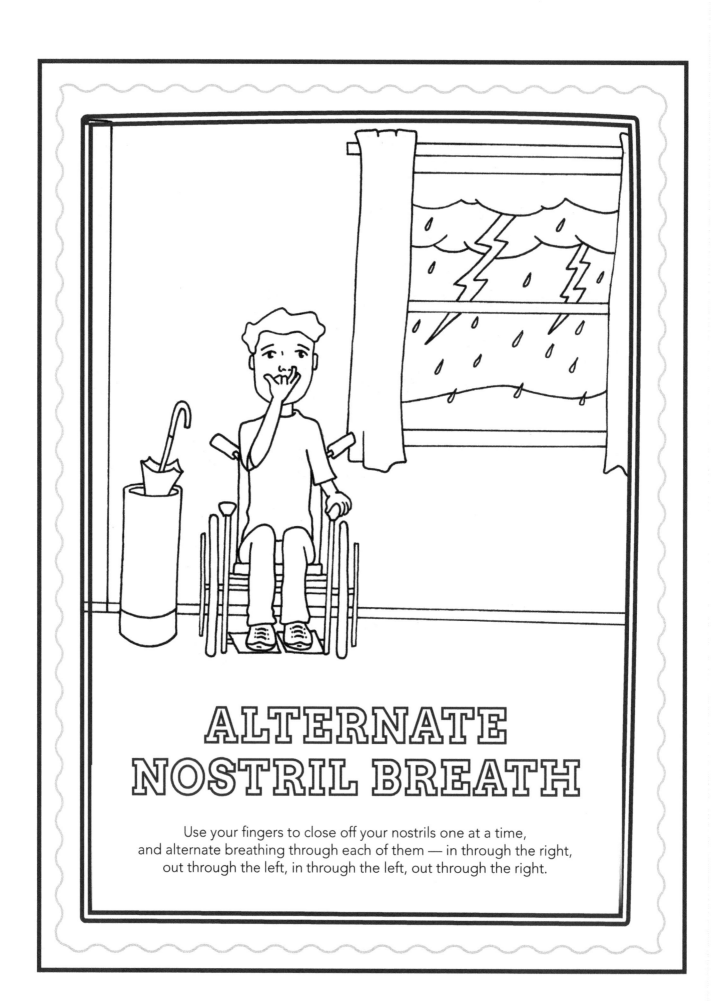

ALTERNATE NOSTRIL BREATH

Use your fingers to close off your nostrils one at a time,
and alternate breathing through each of them — in through the right,
out through the left, in through the left, out through the right.

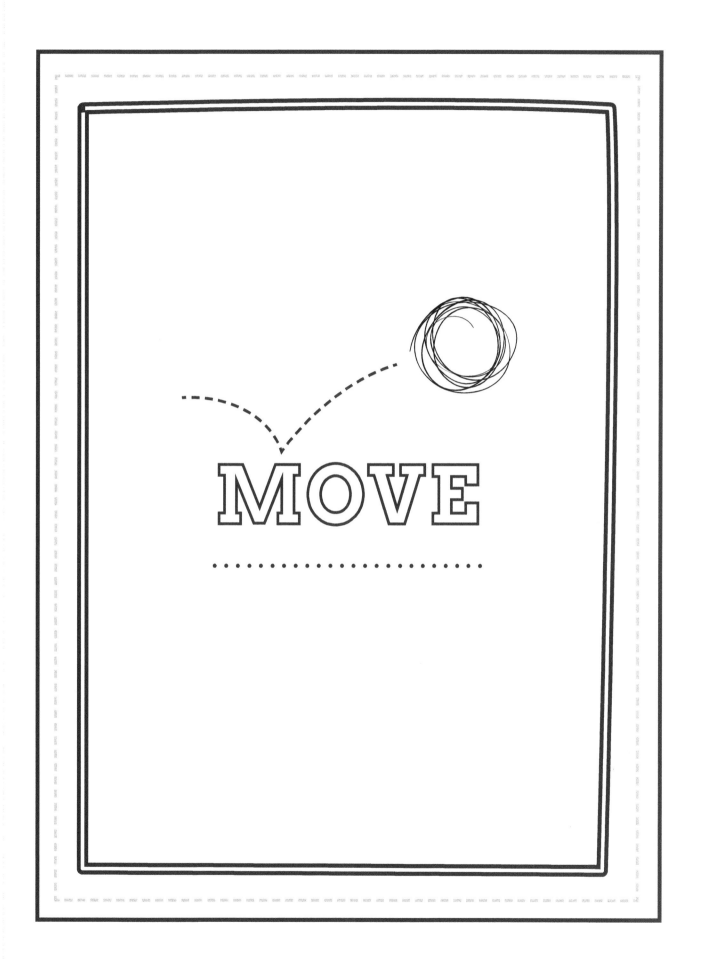

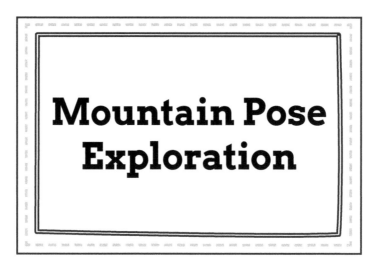

Mountain Pose Exploration

Stand in Mountain Pose, take a few slow breaths, and do a scan of your body. Starting with your feet, and ending with your head, bring your attention to each part of your body and check in with how it is feeling in this pose today.

Now you are going to wake up your body. Bring your attention to your toes and explore how they move. Wiggle them, pick them up, spread them out, and then place them back down. Now move your feet and ankles. Roll them in circles, point and flex your foot, and make any other movements that your feet want to make. Next move your legs and bend your knees. Pick up each knee high, and then bend them as deeply as you can. What other movements can you make with your knees?

Keep moving up your body to your hips and explore how they move. Make big circles with your legs, maybe give each leg a good shake. Make circles with your hips. Continue moving up your body, pausing at each joint to move it any way that feels good. Move your shoulders, arms and hands, your neck. You can even move the muscles in your face (try scrunching your nose, opening and closing your jaw, moving your tongue around and whatever else you can think of).

After you've moved your whole body, come back to Mountain Pose. Take one more scan, going slowly from your feet to your head, of how your body is feeling. Notice if this Mountain Pose feels any different from your first.

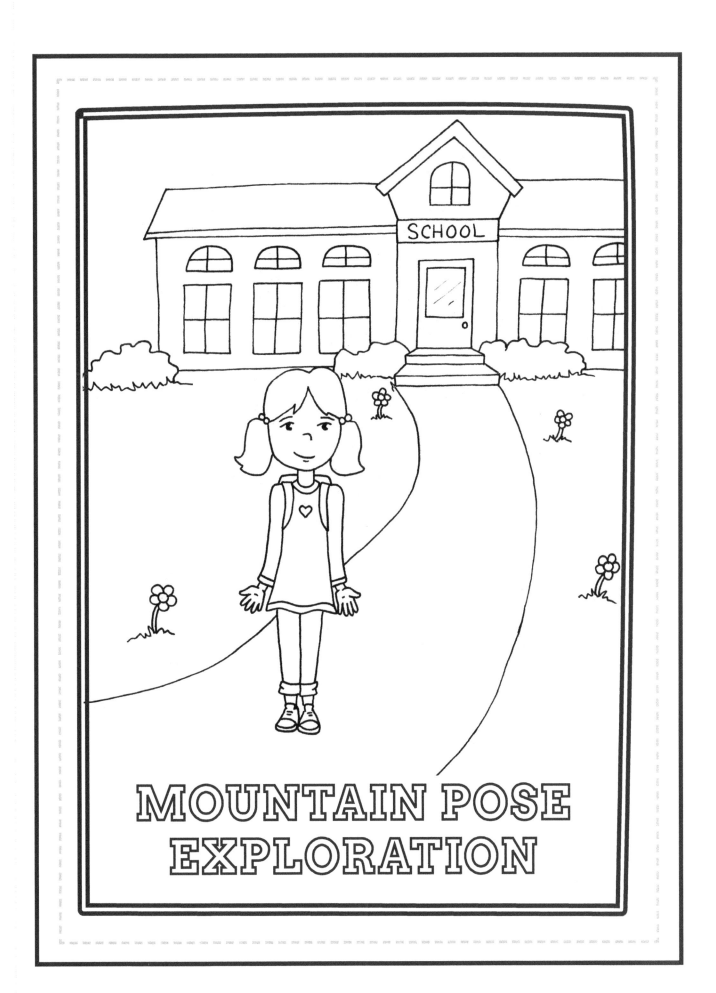

MOUNTAIN POSE
EXPLORATION

Mountain Pose Exploration

Use the space below to write about or draw
what you can experience with each of your senses right now.

How did your body feel in your first
Mountain Pose?

How did your body feel in your second
Mountain Pose, after doing some
movement?

Is there anything else you noticed during this activity?

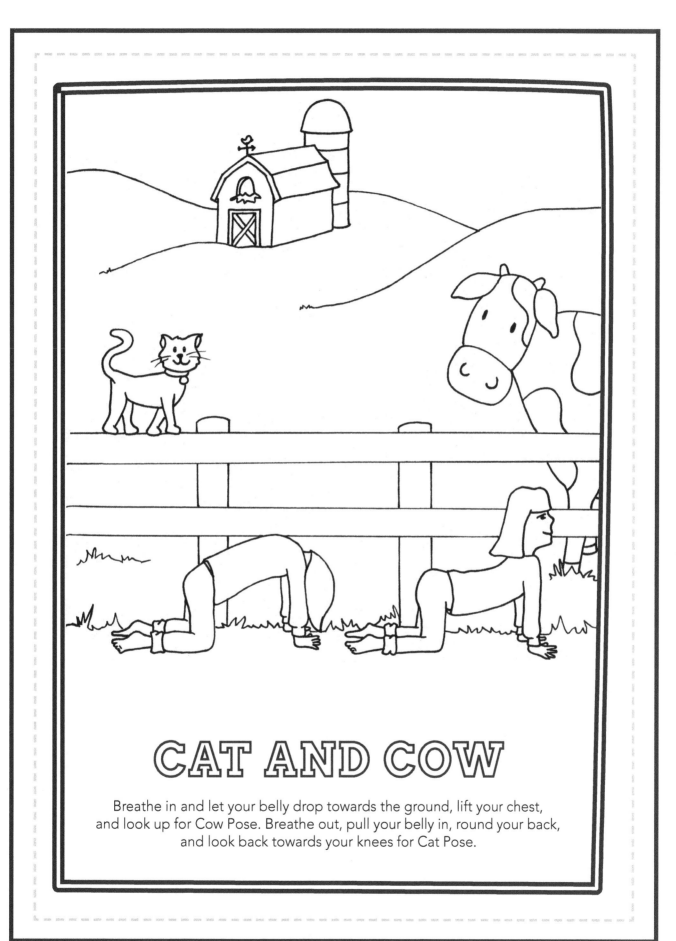

CAT AND COW

Breathe in and let your belly drop towards the ground, lift your chest, and look up for Cow Pose. Breathe out, pull your belly in, round your back, and look back towards your knees for Cat Pose.

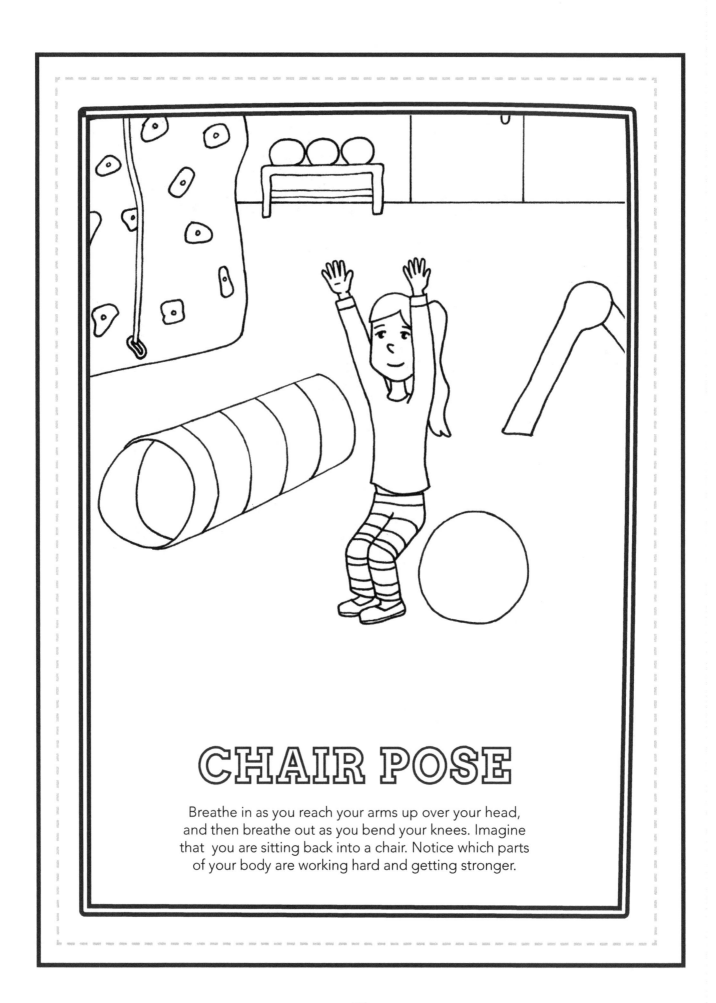

CHAIR POSE

Breathe in as you reach your arms up over your head, and then breathe out as you bend your knees. Imagine that you are sitting back into a chair. Notice which parts of your body are working hard and getting stronger.

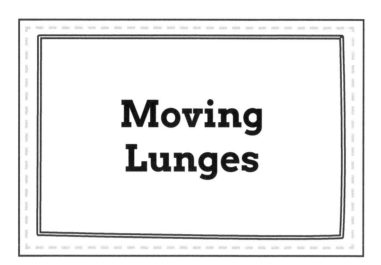

Moving Lunges

Start in Mountain Pose. Lift your right knee up off of the ground and find your balance. Now take a big step backward and place your foot on the floor. Your toes should be pointing straight ahead, with your heel lifted off of the ground.

Bend your front knee deeply (make sure not to bend your knee past your ankle). Keeping your legs steady, reach your arms strongly overhead with your fingers extended. Check to see if you are leaning forward, and if you are, straighten your torso so that it is perpendicular to the ground. Now you are in a lunge. Take a couple of full breaths here in your lunge. Notice how your legs and arms are feeling.

The next time you inhale, slowly straighten your front leg while continuing to reach up with your arms. As you straighten your leg, allow your back heel to lift a little higher off the ground. When it's time to exhale, slowly bend your front knee and press your back heel away from you, lowering your torso straight down. Continue lifting up on your inhale and lowering down on your exhale. Try to keep your upper body moving straight up and down as you bend and straighten your legs, rather then letting it sway forward and backward. Move up and down with your breath for three rounds (or more!) and then repeat on the other side.

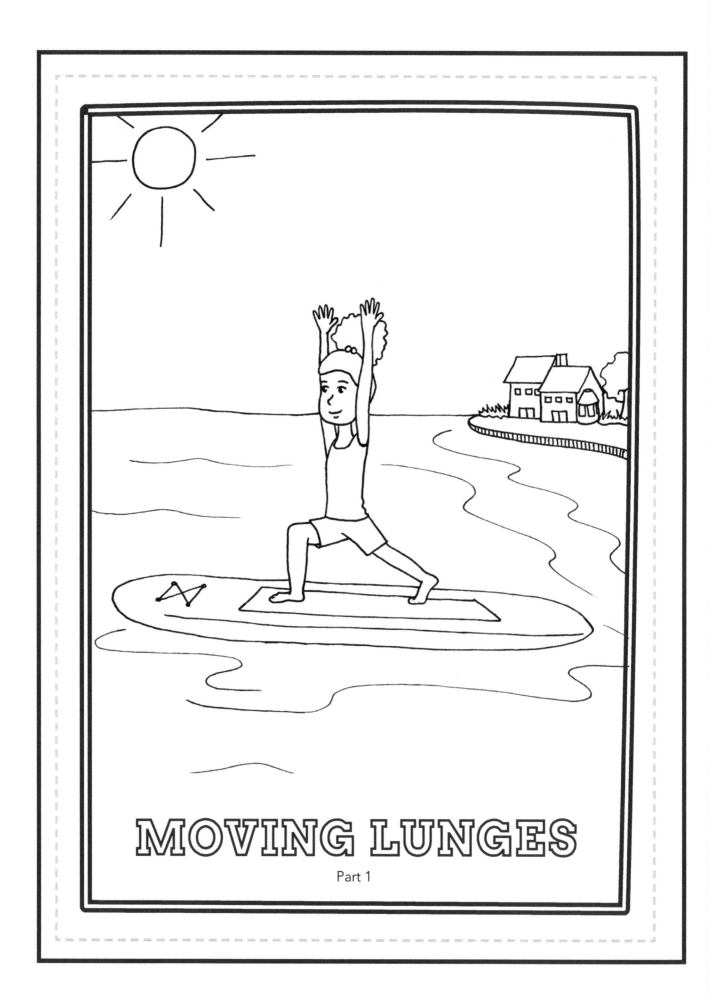

MOVING LUNGES

Part 1

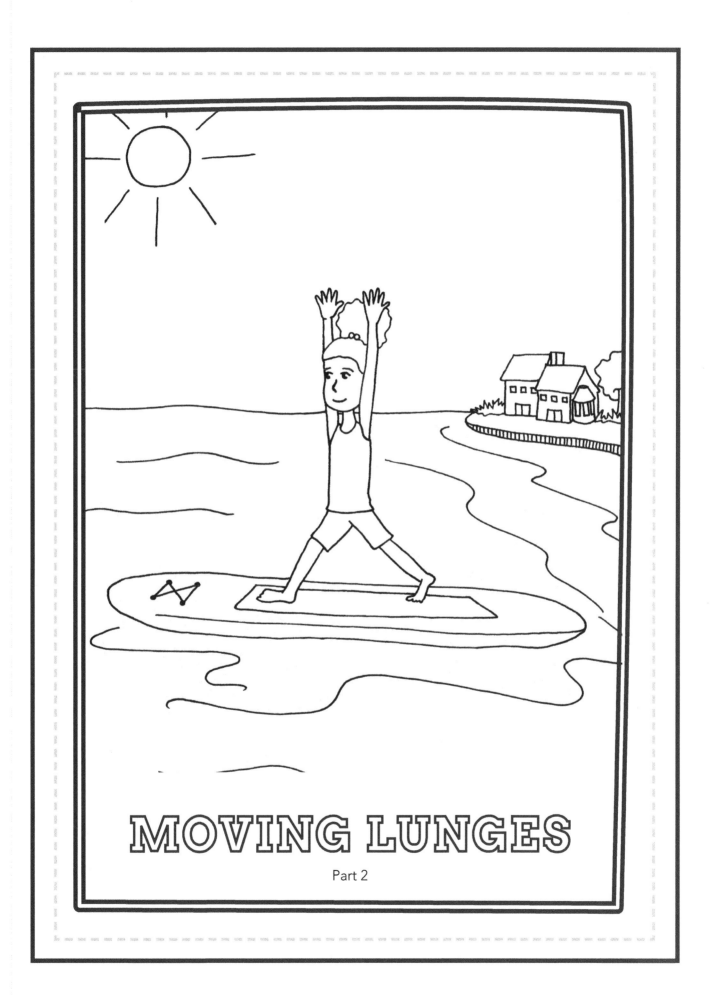

MOVING LUNGES

Part 2

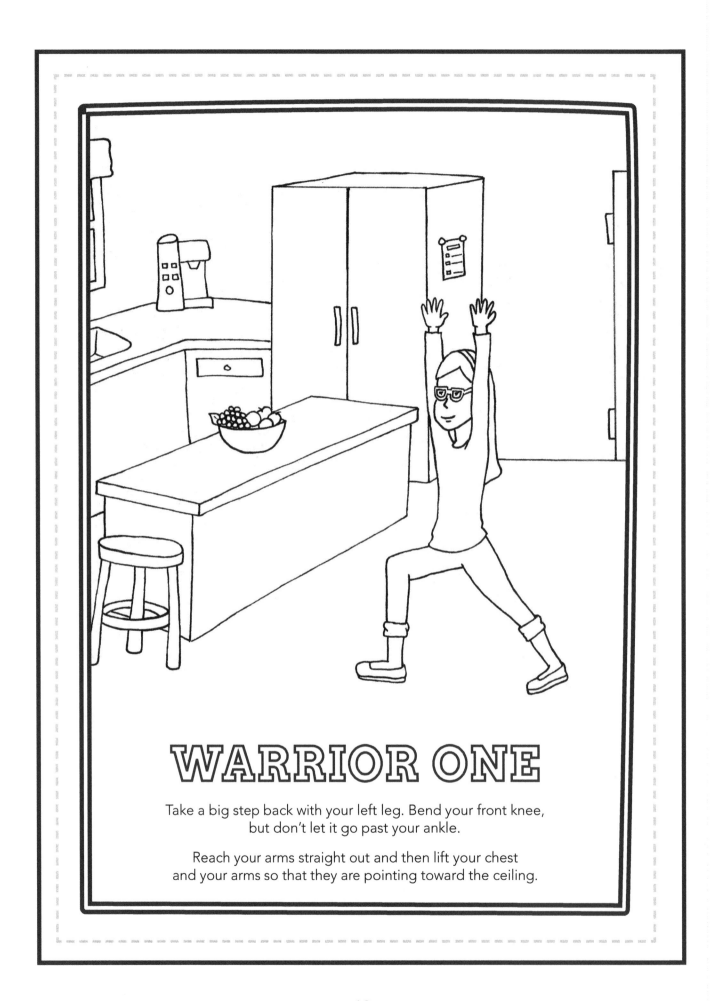

WARRIOR ONE

Take a big step back with your left leg. Bend your front knee,
but don't let it go past your ankle.

Reach your arms straight out and then lift your chest
and your arms so that they are pointing toward the ceiling.

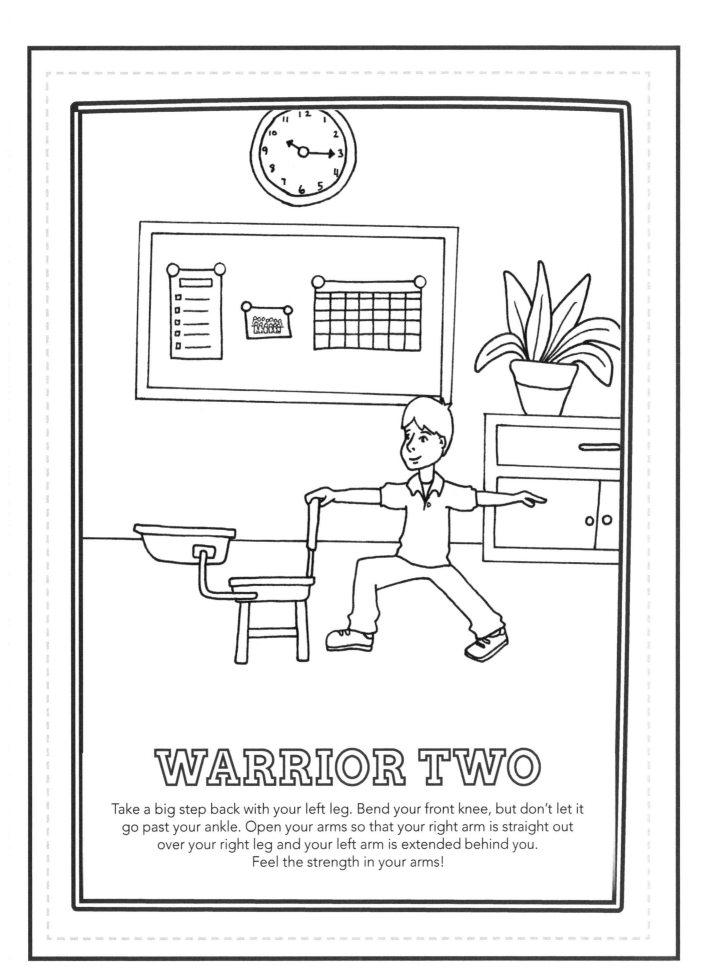

WARRIOR TWO

Take a big step back with your left leg. Bend your front knee, but don't let it
go past your ankle. Open your arms so that your right arm is straight out
over your right leg and your left arm is extended behind you.
Feel the strength in your arms!

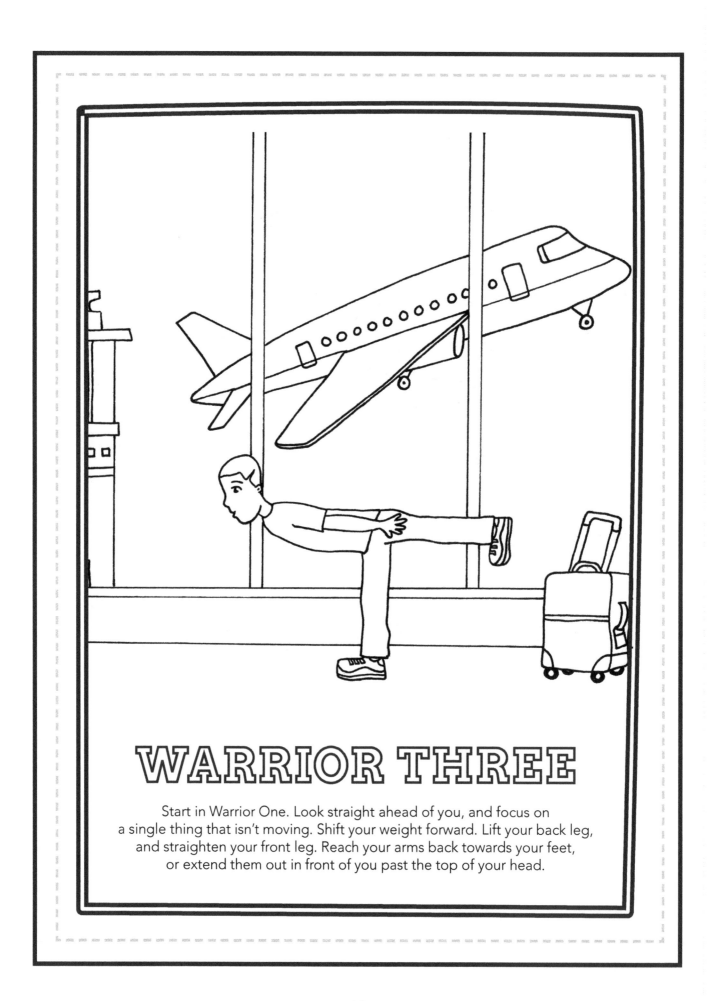

WARRIOR THREE

Start in Warrior One. Look straight ahead of you, and focus on
a single thing that isn't moving. Shift your weight forward. Lift your back leg,
and straighten your front leg. Reach your arms back towards your feet,
or extend them out in front of you past the top of your head.

The Warriors Exploration

What is a warrior? Can you be a warrior without hurting anyone? How?

Is there anyone in your life that is a warrior for you?

Is there anyone or anything that you are a warrior for?

What are some qualities that a good warrior needs to have, especially a peaceful warrior?

Try practicing the three Warrior Poses, and with each one, say outloud the qualities you've listed above. For example in Warrior 1 say "I am strong," and then move into Warrior 2 saying "I am _____ ; and Warrior 3 saying "I am _____ ."
Try different combinations of qualities and see what it feels like.

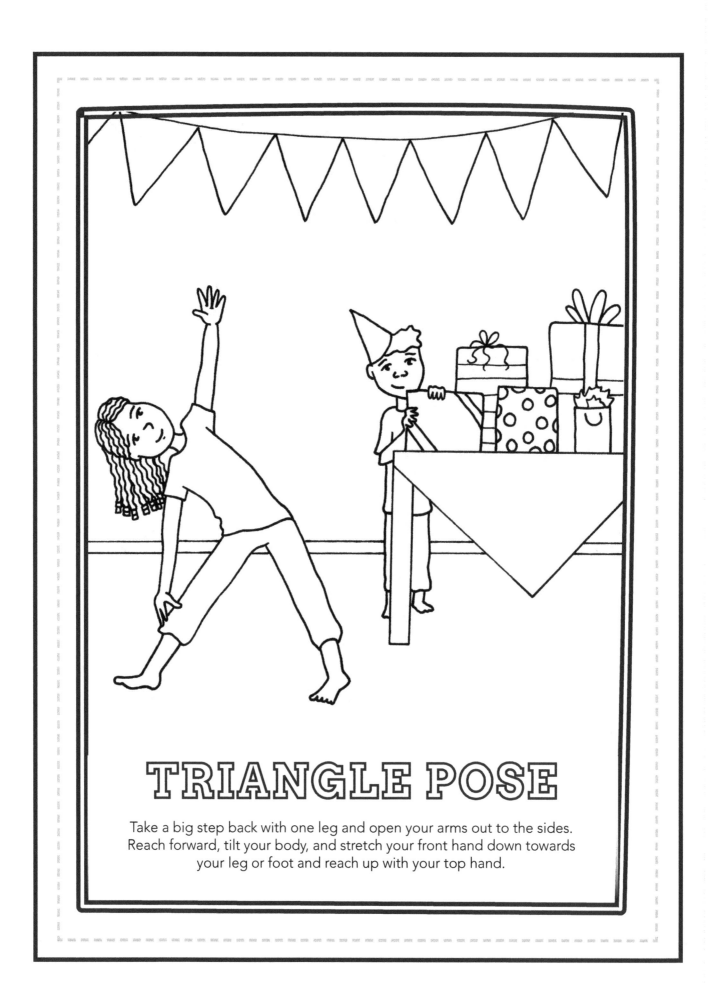

TRIANGLE POSE

Take a big step back with one leg and open your arms out to the sides.
Reach forward, tilt your body, and stretch your front hand down towards
your leg or foot and reach up with your top hand.

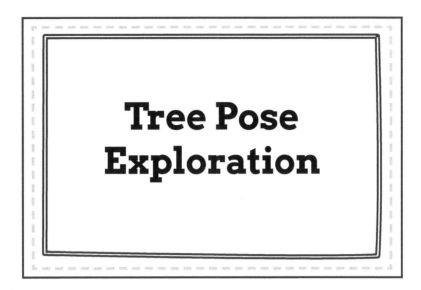

Tree Pose Exploration

Begin standing in Mountain Pose. Find a place to rest your gaze that is straight out in front of you. Keep staring at that spot to help you balance. Slowly lift your right foot up off of the ground. Bend your knee and turn it out to the side, so that you can place the sole of your right foot on the inside of your left calf. You can also lift your foot to the inside of your thigh, but make sure not to place it on the side of your knee.

Try to relax the foot of your standing leg. Notice if you are curling up your toes, and if so wiggle them a little bit. Imagine your standing leg growing roots deep into the ground to hold you steady. Press your foot into your leg, and your leg back into your foot. Lift your arms overhead like branches reaching for the sun.

When you are ready to switch sides, turn your right knee to the front, pause, and then slowly lower it down. Then practice Tree Pose with your left leg.

Now practice Tree Pose again, but this time, try an experiment. While you're holding the pose, look up, then right, then left, then down…move your eyes quickly and notice what happens in your body. Now try looking at something that is moving, such as leaves blowing on trees, cars going by, or anything else that has a bit of movement to it. How do you feel? Finally try closing your eyes, and see what happens to your balance.

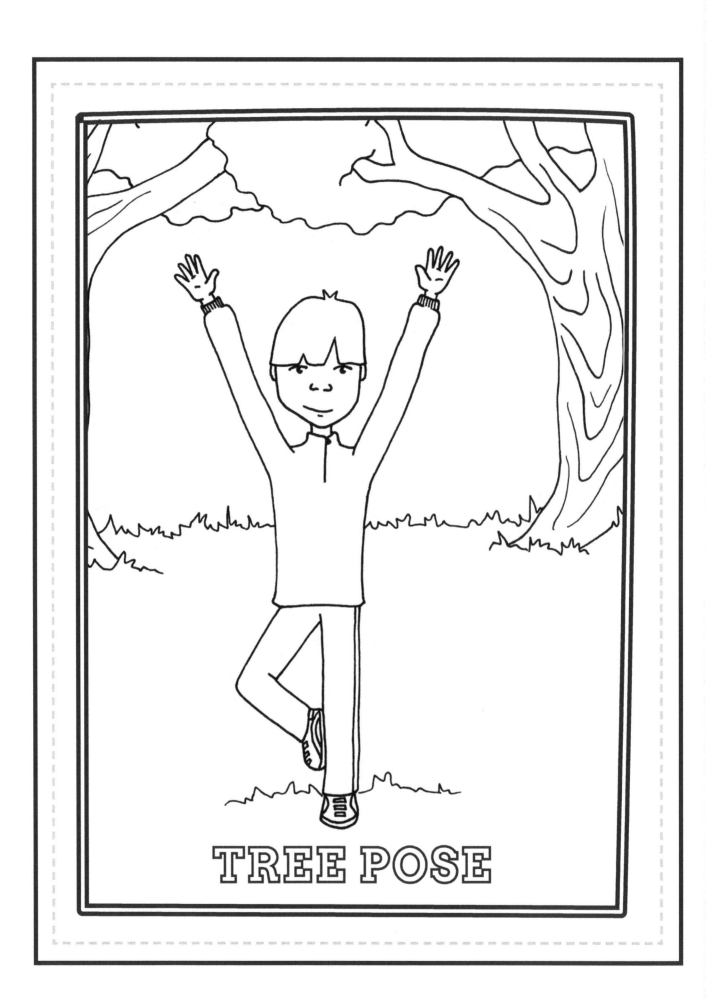

TREE POSE

Tree Pose
Exploration

How did you feel in Tree Pose?

_____

_____

_____

What happended when:

You looked around?   _____

_____

_____

You looked at something that was moving? _____

_____

_____

You closed your eyes? _____

_____

_____

Did you notice anything else?

_____

_____

_____

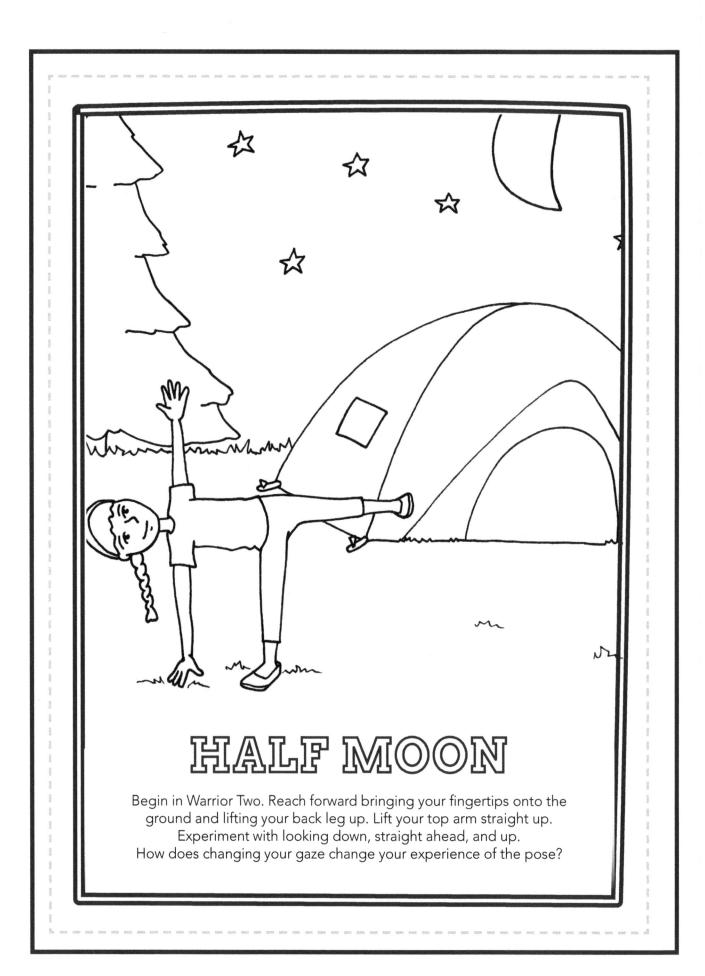

HALF MOON

Begin in Warrior Two. Reach forward bringing your fingertips onto the
ground and lifting your back leg up. Lift your top arm straight up.
Experiment with looking down, straight ahead, and up.
How does changing your gaze change your experience of the pose?

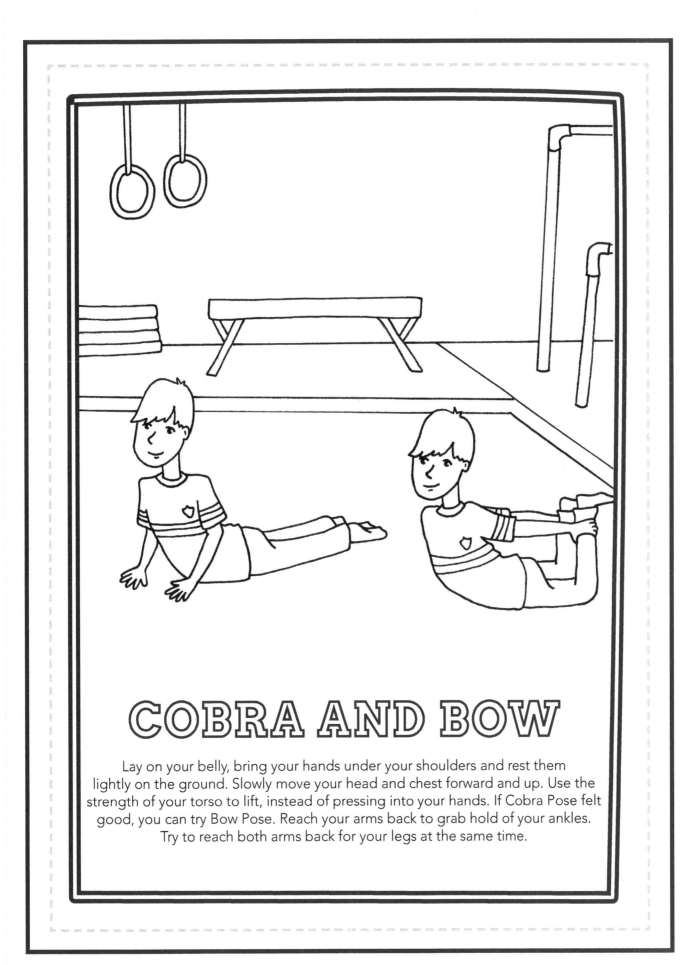

COBRA AND BOW

Lay on your belly, bring your hands under your shoulders and rest them lightly on the ground. Slowly move your head and chest forward and up. Use the strength of your torso to lift, instead of pressing into your hands. If Cobra Pose felt good, you can try Bow Pose. Reach your arms back to grab hold of your ankles. Try to reach both arms back for your legs at the same time.

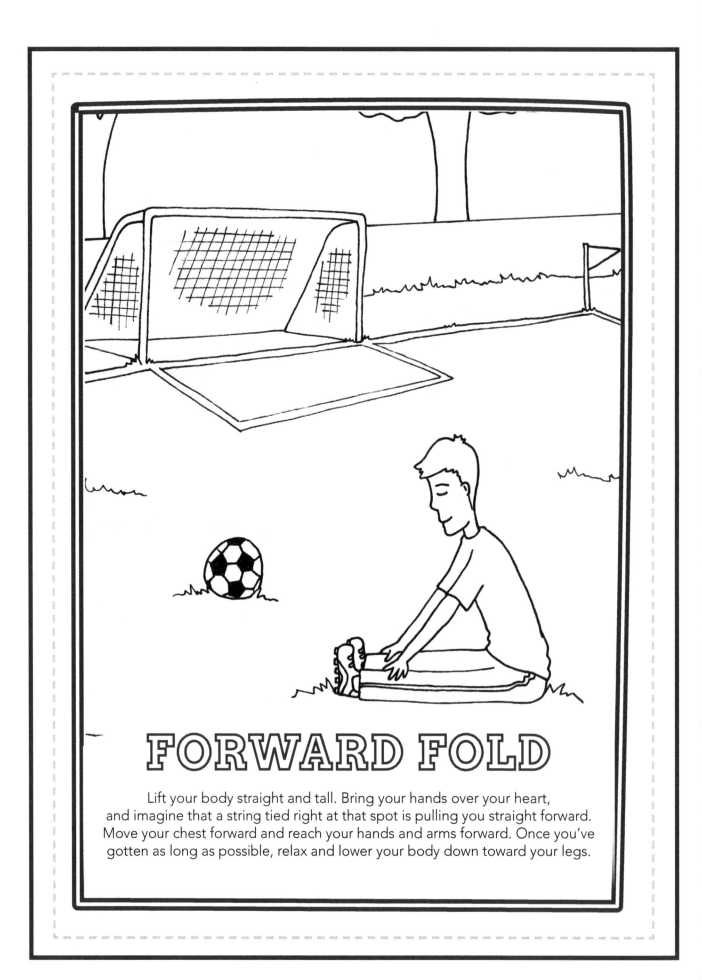

FORWARD FOLD

Lift your body straight and tall. Bring your hands over your heart,
and imagine that a string tied right at that spot is pulling you straight forward.
Move your chest forward and reach your hands and arms forward. Once you've
gotten as long as possible, relax and lower your body down toward your legs.

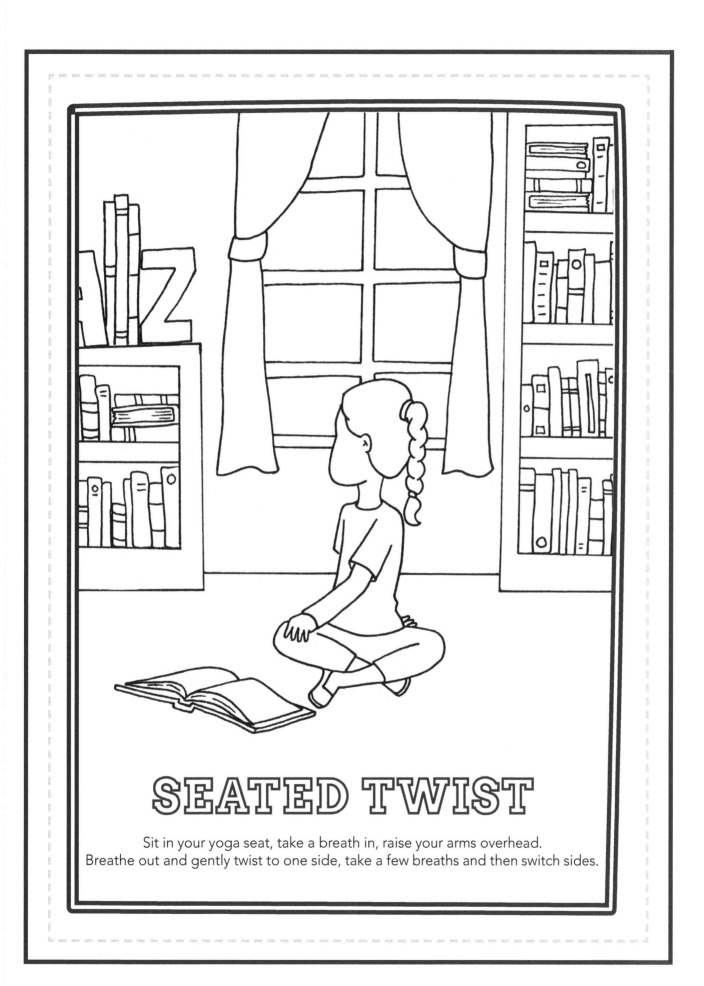

SEATED TWIST

Sit in your yoga seat, take a breath in, raise your arms overhead.
Breathe out and gently twist to one side, take a few breaths and then switch sides.

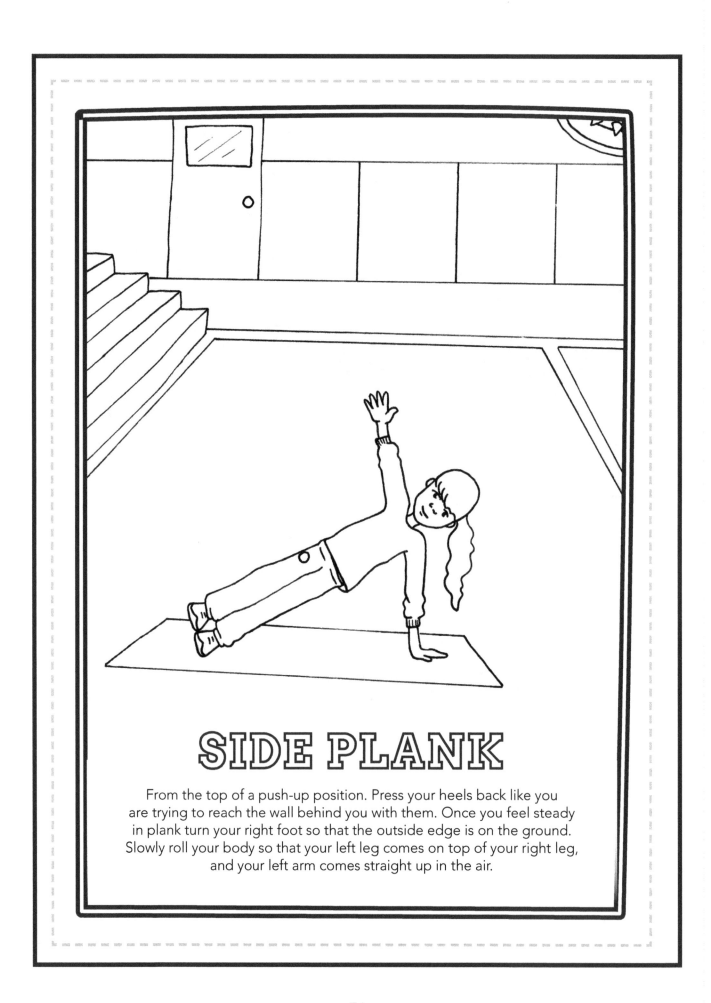

SIDE PLANK

From the top of a push-up position. Press your heels back like you are trying to reach the wall behind you with them. Once you feel steady in plank turn your right foot so that the outside edge is on the ground. Slowly roll your body so that your left leg comes on top of your right leg, and your left arm comes straight up in the air.

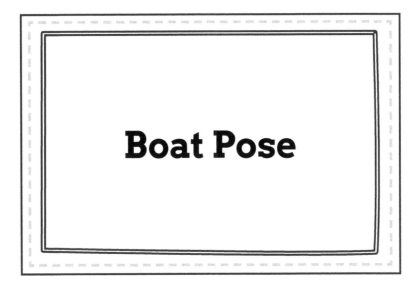

Boat Pose

Sit tall with your knees bent and your feet flat on the ground. Lightly hold on to the back of your thighs with your hands. Lean your body back until you feel the muscles in your core (your belly and your back) starting to work. Hold your body steady, and then lift your feet, bringing your shins parallel with the ground. Find your balance and take a few steadying breaths. Use each inhalation to sit up a little bit taller. If you feel steady, experiment with straightening your legs and reaching your arms out in front of you.

Notice what parts of your body are working hard in this pose. Are there any parts of your body that can relax? Any parts that are stretching? Experiment with lifting your legs higher, and lowering them down closer to the ground. How does changing your leg position change the way your body feels?

When you're ready to finish, bring your feet to the ground, sit up, and take a few slow breaths.

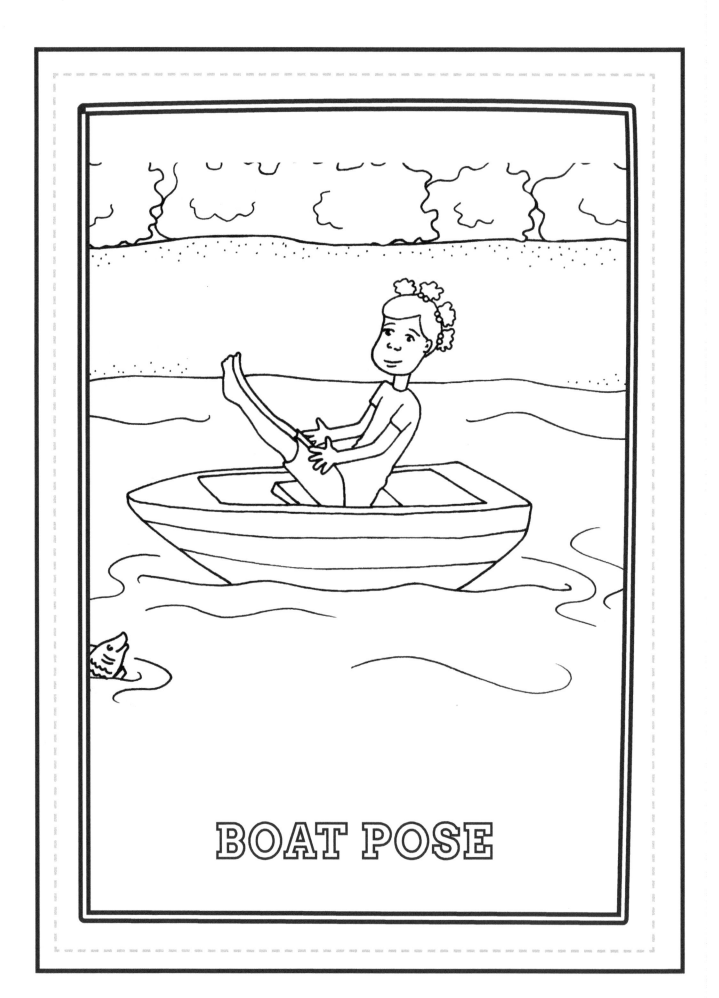

BOAT POSE

BOAT POSE
EXPLORATION

In Boat Pose you are using your body's strength and flexibility
at the same time. Let's explore how that is working.

What parts of your body are working hard
and getting stronger in this pose?

What parts of your body
are stretching in this pose?

Are any parts of your body relaxing in Boat Pose?
If not, try experimenting. Can any part of your body relax?

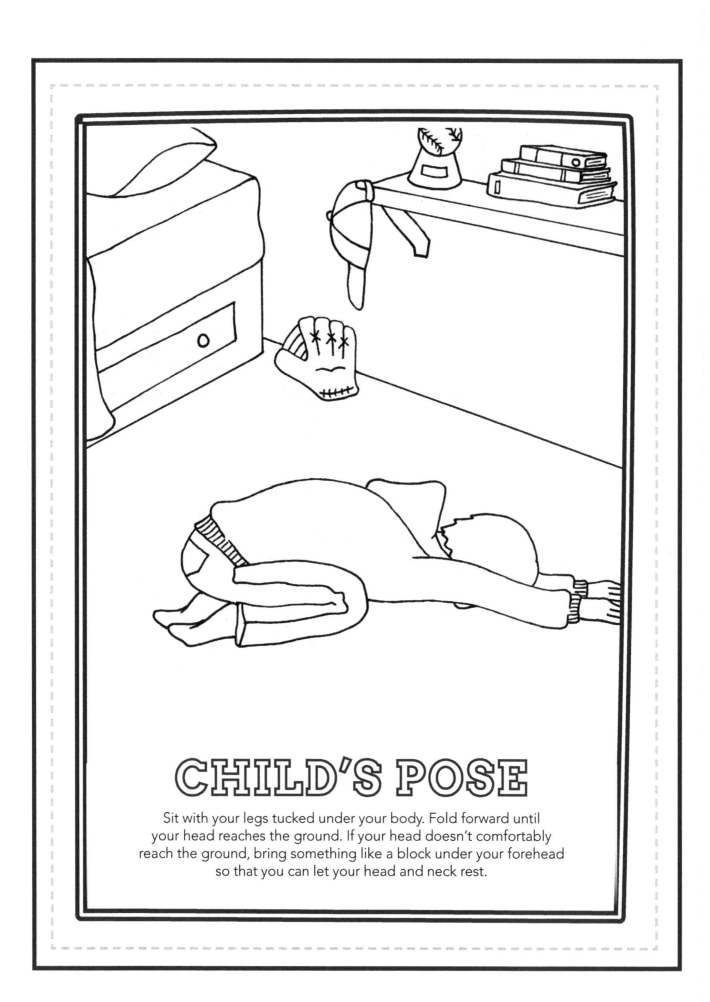

CHILD'S POSE

Sit with your legs tucked under your body. Fold forward until your head reaches the ground. If your head doesn't comfortably reach the ground, bring something like a block under your forehead so that you can let your head and neck rest.

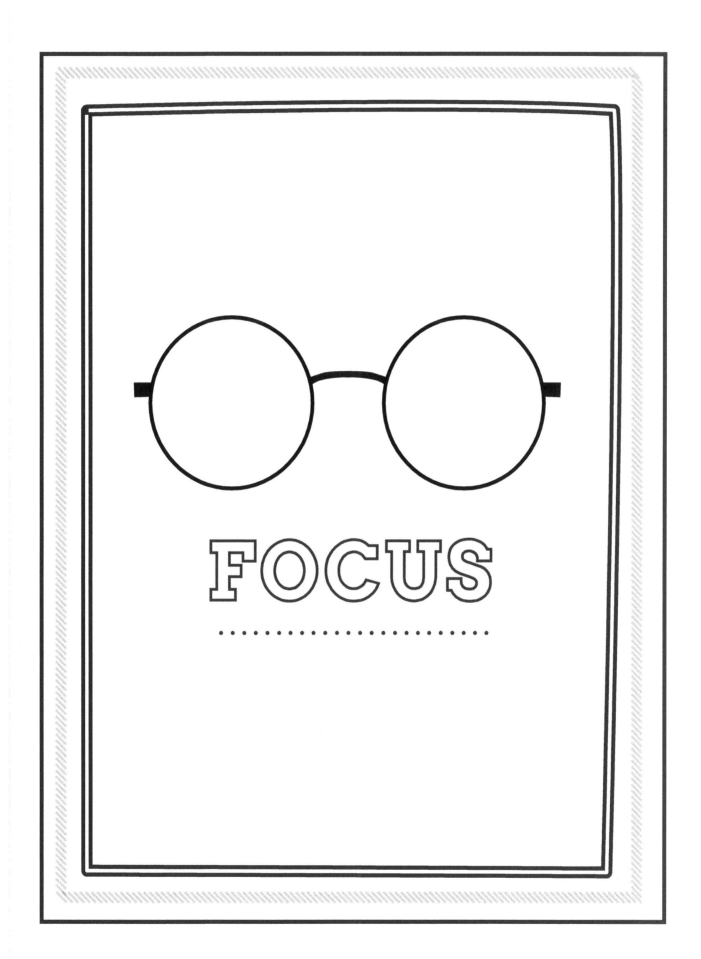

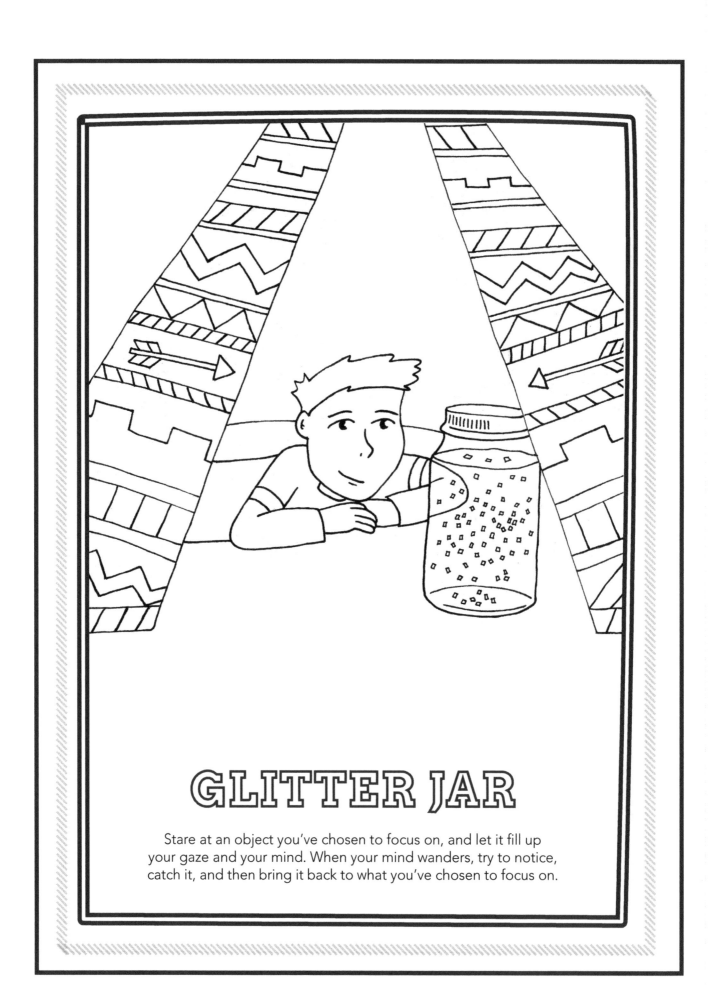

GLITTER JAR

Stare at an object you've chosen to focus on, and let it fill up your gaze and your mind. When your mind wanders, try to notice, catch it, and then bring it back to what you've chosen to focus on.

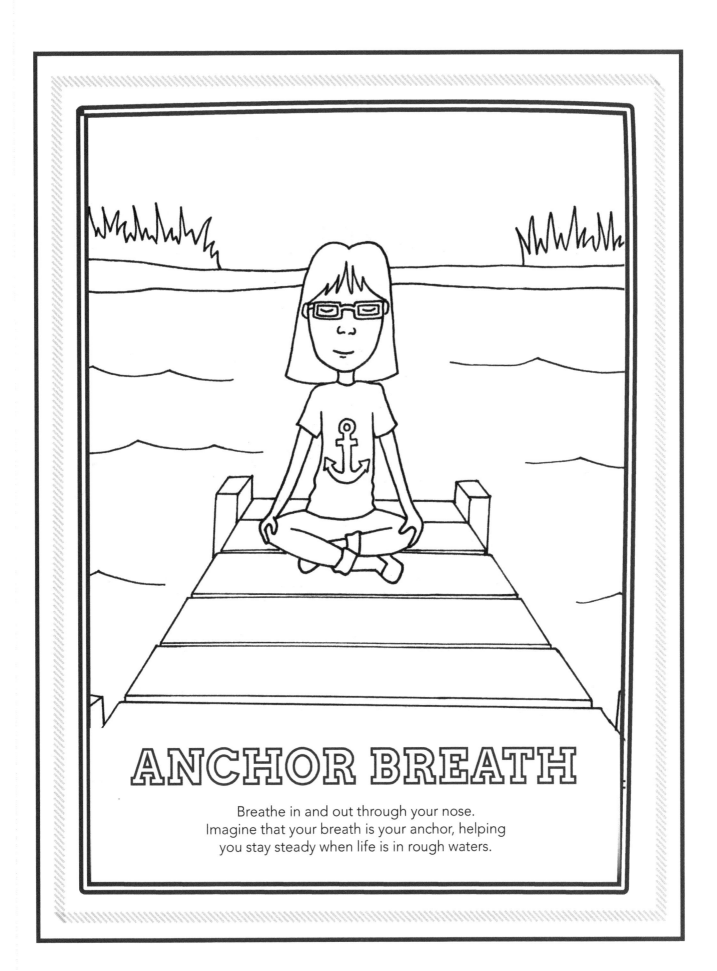

ANCHOR BREATH

Breathe in and out through your nose.
Imagine that your breath is your anchor, helping
you stay steady when life is in rough waters.

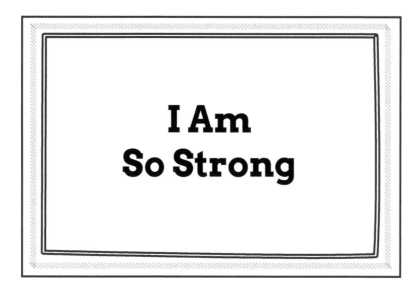

**I Am
So Strong**

Combine the movement of your hands with a powerful statement or affirmation towards yourself. Begin by connecting your thumb to your pointer finger for "I," your thumb and middle finger for "am," your thumb and ring finger for "so," and thumb and pinkie for "strong."

Use enough pressure to feel the connection your fingers are making. Begin slowly, saying "I am so strong" using both hands simultaneously, and as you feel more comfortable you can go a bit faster. Experiment with what it feels like to say the statement out loud, verses saying it silently to yourself. Continue for as long as you would like, about 30 seconds is great to start, and when you are finished take a few slow breaths before you go on with your day.

You can always try out other statements as well, such as "I'm Full of Love," "I Am In Charge," "I Can Do This" or anything else you think you need to hear.

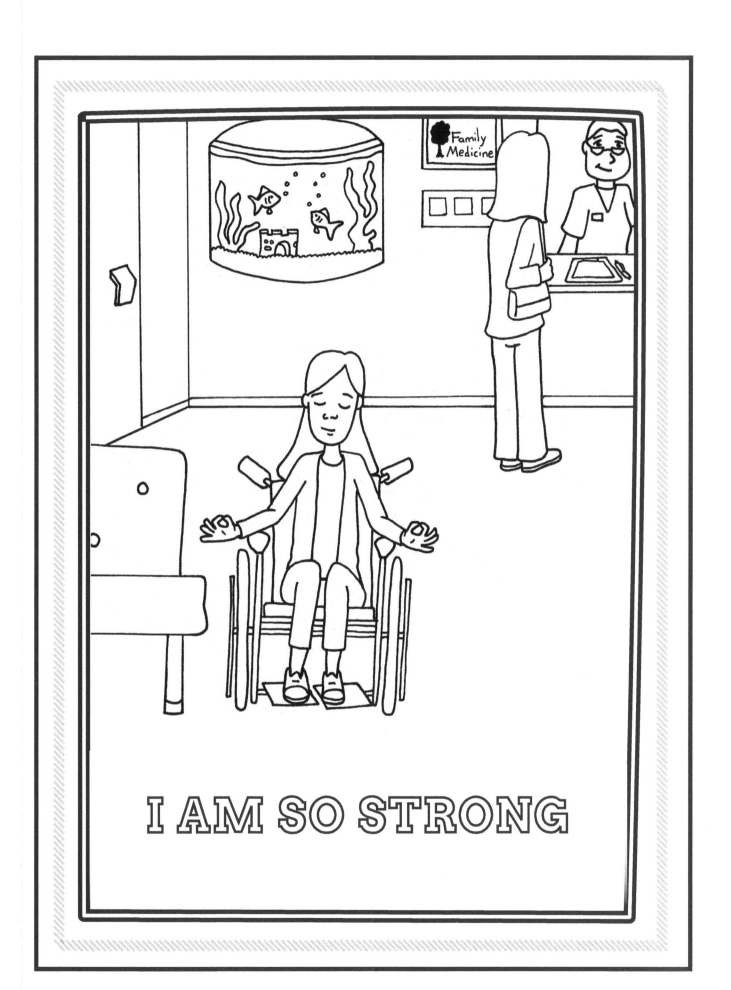

Create Your Own Affirmation

What are the things you really need to hear today? Imagine that you're your own best friend, and create some power statements to help you feel like your best self. Try using them with the hand movements you learned in the "I AM SO STRONG" activity.

(*) _____

(*) _____

(*) _____

(*) _____

(*) _____

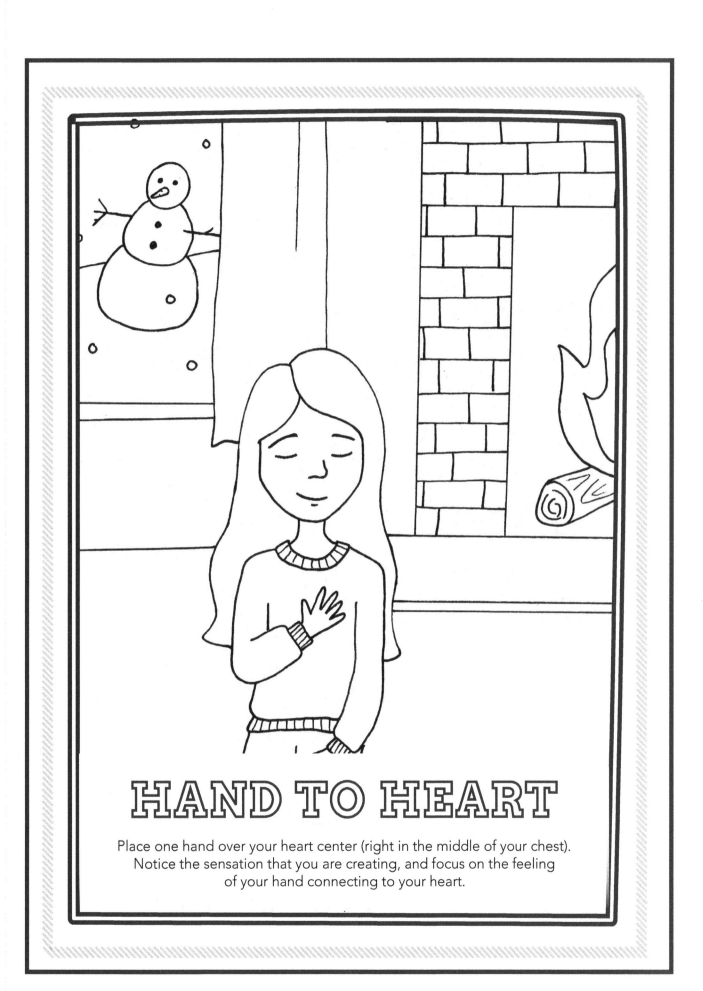

HAND TO HEART

Place one hand over your heart center (right in the middle of your chest).
Notice the sensation that you are creating, and focus on the feeling
of your hand connecting to your heart.

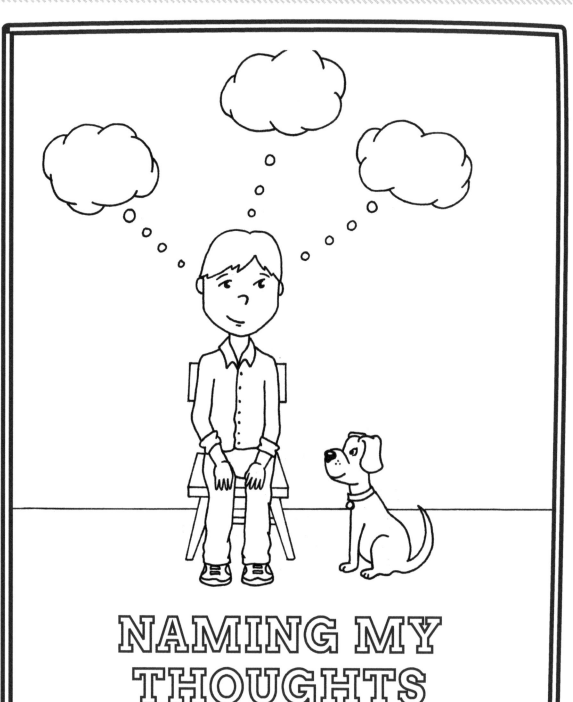

NAMING MY THOUGHTS

Sit quietly, and as thoughts pop into your head, practice naming
your thoughts. If an idea pops in, silently say "ideas." If you find yourself
remembering something, silently say "memory" and if you start thinking
about all the things you have to do you might say "planning" or "worrying."
Try writing the kinds of thoughts you're having in the bubbles of the picture.

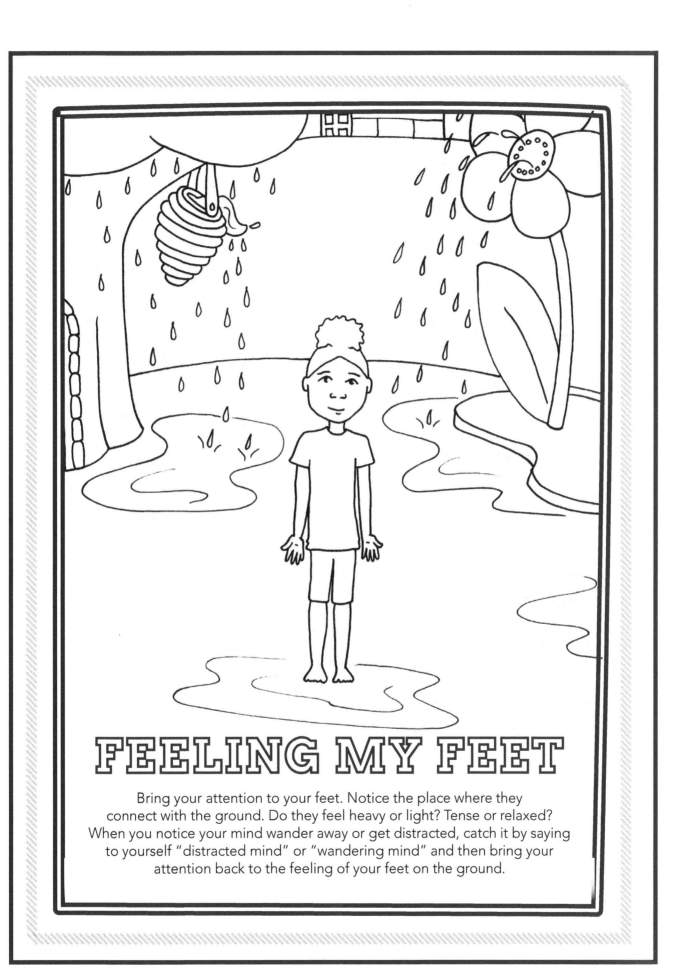

FEELING MY FEET

Bring your attention to your feet. Notice the place where they connect with the ground. Do they feel heavy or light? Tense or relaxed? When you notice your mind wander away or get distracted, catch it by saying to yourself "distracted mind" or "wandering mind" and then bring your attention back to the feeling of your feet on the ground.

Expanding Energy Meditation

Sit on your mat, with your body tall and relaxed. Take a few full breaths to settle your body and your mind, and then close your eyes. Bring your hands together and begin to rub your palms vigorously. Continue to rub faster and faster until your hands feel warm, then slowly stop rubbing and keep your palms together.

Imagine that between your hands is a very tiny but very bright and strong ball of light and energy. As you take a full breath in, very, very slowly separate your hands and imagine that ball of light growing and expanding, filling your hands with energy.

When you are ready to breathe out, gently and slowly push your hands back together, squeezing that ball of light until it gets very small.

Continue expanding your energy ball as you breathe in and squeezing it together as you breathe out, keeping the rest of your body as still as you can. Try practicing Expanding Energy Meditation for about two minutes the first time you try it, and then a little bit longer each time after that.

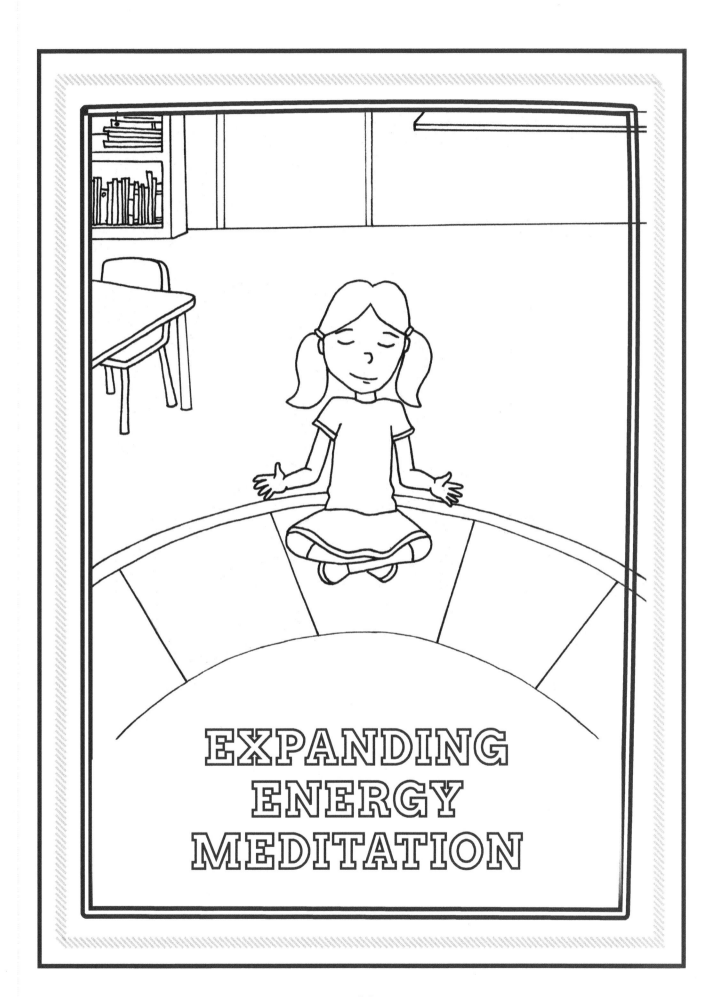

EXPANDING
ENERGY
MEDITATION

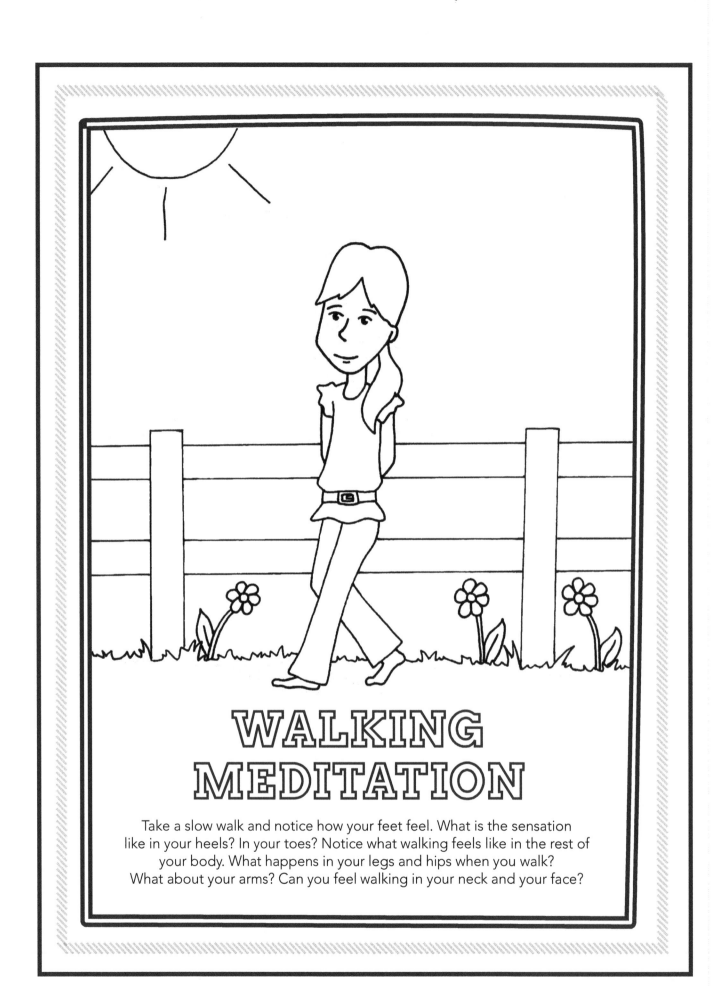

WALKING MEDITATION

Take a slow walk and notice how your feet feel. What is the sensation like in your heels? In your toes? Notice what walking feels like in the rest of your body. What happens in your legs and hips when you walk? What about your arms? Can you feel walking in your neck and your face?

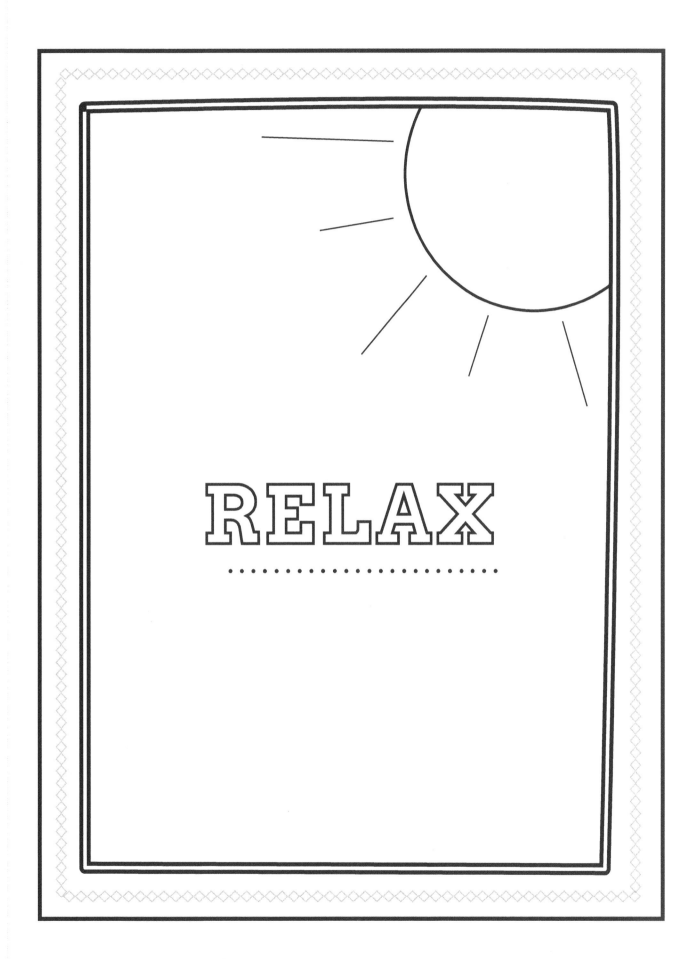

RELAX

Tense
and Let Go

Begin laying down on your mat or another comfortable place. Spend a few moments here just paying attention to your breath and getting settled. Now you are going to bring your attention to each part of your body, starting with your toes and moving all the way up to your head. As you think about each part of your body, you will tense the muscles in that body part, and then let them relax, until you have invited your whole body to relax.

First think about your toes. Scrunch them up as tight as you can, hold them there for a second or two, and then let them rest. Now tense up both of your feet, and when you let them relax, imagine that they are very, very heavy.

Now tighten the muscles in your calves and around your knees. Try counting to five before letting them relax. Next squeeze all of the muscles in your legs. You might find yourself squeezing so hard that your legs lift off of the ground a tiny bit. After a few seconds, let all of the muscles in your legs relax, and feel your legs settle comfortably into the ground. Next pull your belly button in for a few seconds, and then let your belly get very soft. Relax your back into the floor.

Scrunch your shoulders up to your ears, then after a few seconds relax them down. Make your hands into very tight fists, and squeeze all of the muscles in your arms. Just like your legs, you may find that your arms come off of the ground a little, and that is great. Now relax your arms and your hands, letting them rest by your sides with your palms facing up.

Close your eyes very tightly, scrunch up your nose, and squeeze your lips together. Hold your face in this tensed position for a few seconds, and then let your whole face relax. Take a big breath in and, when you exhale, let out a deep sigh through your mouth.

Now take a minute to pay attention to your whole body. If you notice any part that still feels uncomfortable or isn't very relaxed, go ahead and tense it up, then let go, until you've relaxed each part of you. Once your body is relaxed, rest for as long as you'd like.

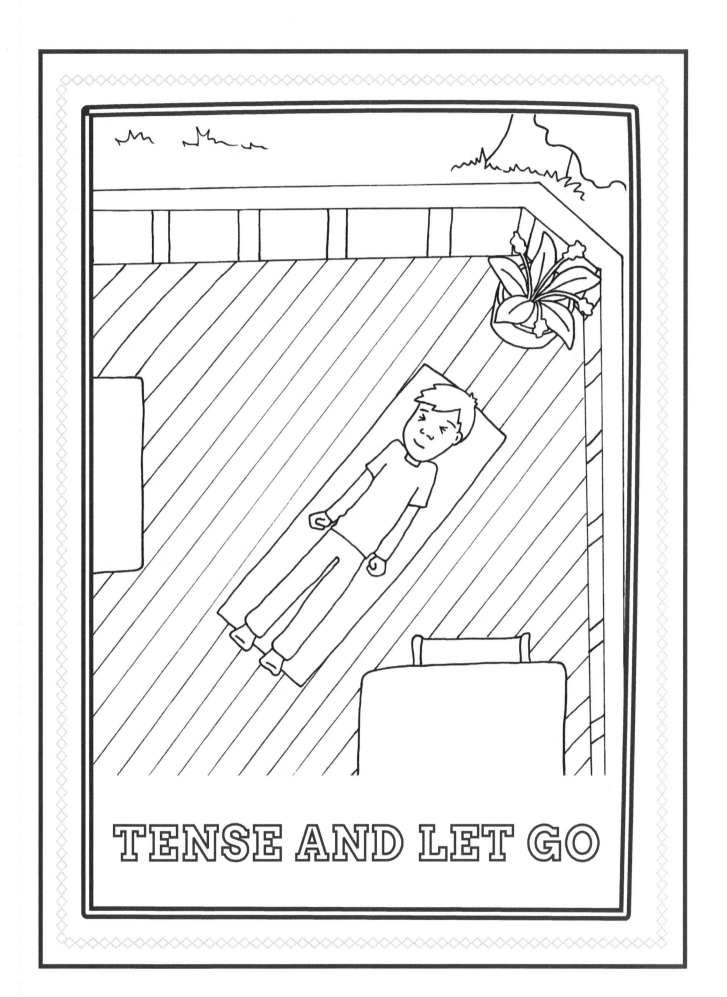

TENSE AND LET GO

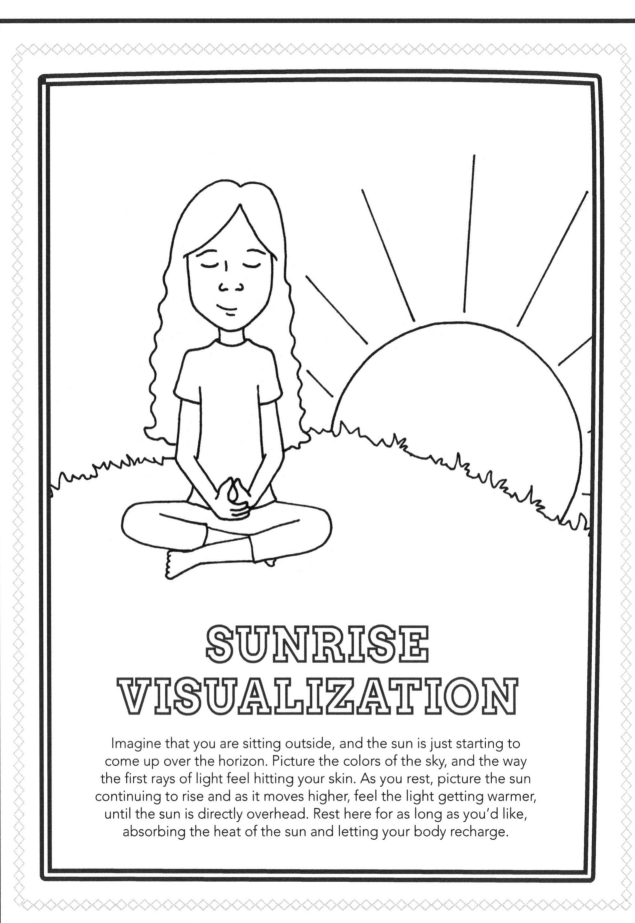

SUNRISE VISUALIZATION

Imagine that you are sitting outside, and the sun is just starting to come up over the horizon. Picture the colors of the sky, and the way the first rays of light feel hitting your skin. As you rest, picture the sun continuing to rise and as it moves higher, feel the light getting warmer, until the sun is directly overhead. Rest here for as long as you'd like, absorbing the heat of the sun and letting your body recharge.

Sunrise
Visualization

Draw your own sunrise here

Mountain Top Visualization

Sit up tall on the floor or a chair. Close your eyes or rest them in one place. Imagine that you are sitting outside, looking up at a tall mountain. Now imagine that you are getting ready to climb this mountain. Imagine standing and beginning to walk uphill. How are your legs feeling? Take a full breath in and notice how the mountain air smells. Look around. Are you in the woods? Are there flowers? Birds? What else can you see?

As you continue to climb, the path gets steeper, and you have to work much harder. Soon you have to use your hands also, and your body is working very hard. Imagine how your muscles are feeling. What is happening to your breathing? Pause in your climb and look around. What can you see now?

As you get close to the top of the mountain, notice how you are feeling. Imagine reaching the very top. You've done it! Stand at the top of the mountain and appreciate the hard work you did to get here. Look out over the surrounding land.

When you're ready, lay down on your yoga mat (and imagine laying down on the earth at the top of the mountain). Imagine how good this rest would feel after your long climb, your hard work. Let your body sink into the ground. Notice the feeling of the mountain air on your body, and the steady support of the earth underneath you. Rest here for as long as you'd like.

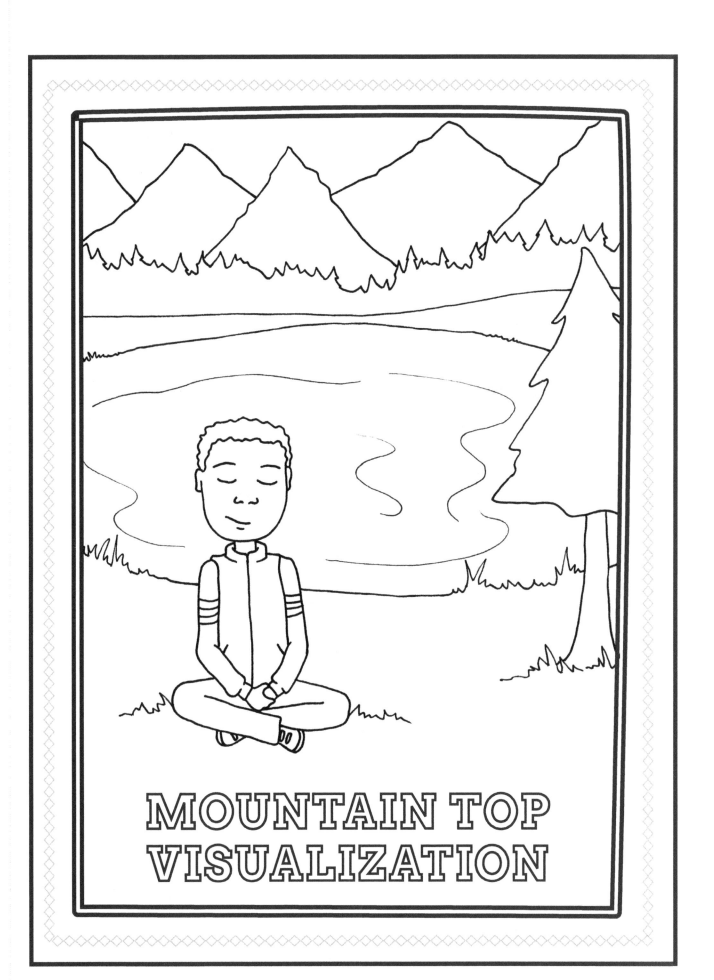

MOUNTAIN TOP
VISUALIZATION

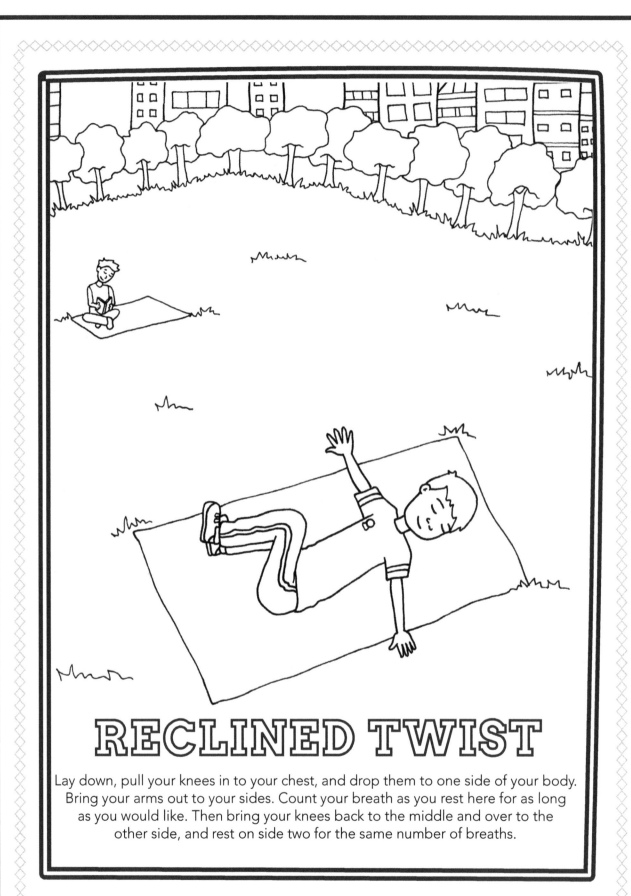

RECLINED TWIST

Lay down, pull your knees in to your chest, and drop them to one side of your body. Bring your arms out to your sides. Count your breath as you rest here for as long as you would like. Then bring your knees back to the middle and over to the other side, and rest on side two for the same number of breaths.

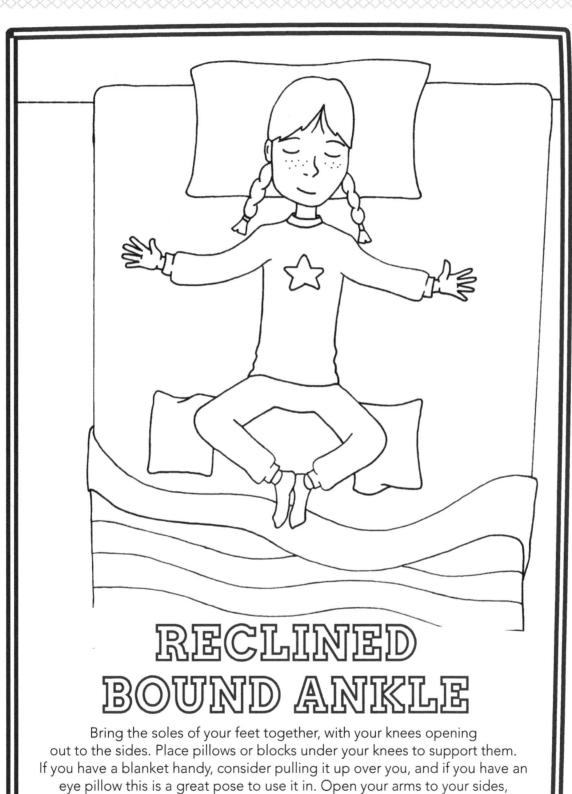

RECLINED
BOUND ANKLE

Bring the soles of your feet together, with your knees opening
out to the sides. Place pillows or blocks under your knees to support them.
If you have a blanket handy, consider pulling it up over you, and if you have an
eye pillow this is a great pose to use it in. Open your arms to your sides,
with your palms facing up, and rest as long as you want.

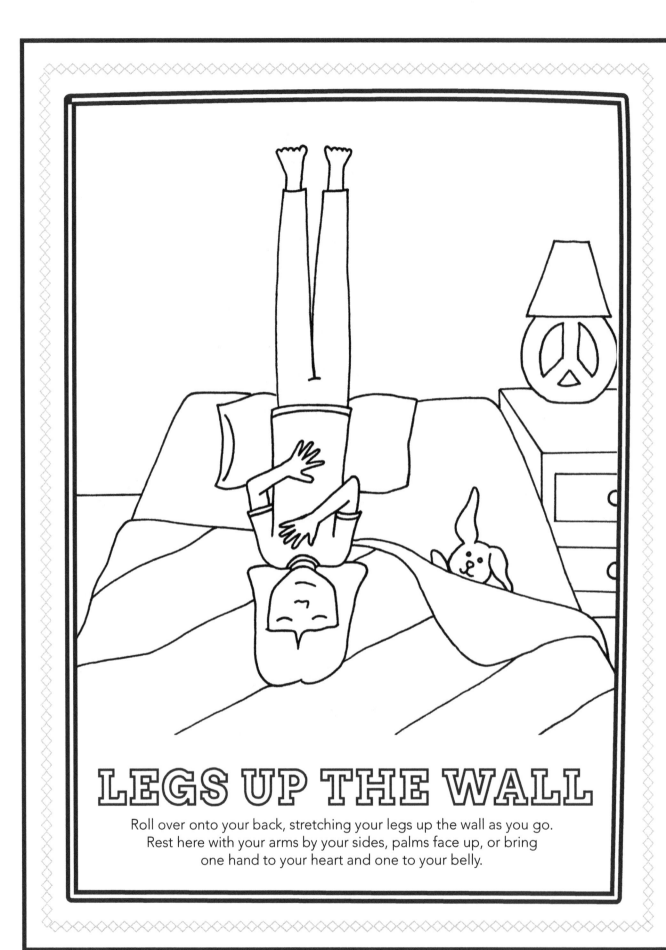

LEGS UP THE WALL

Roll over onto your back, stretching your legs up the wall as you go.
Rest here with your arms by your sides, palms face up, or bring
one hand to your heart and one to your belly.

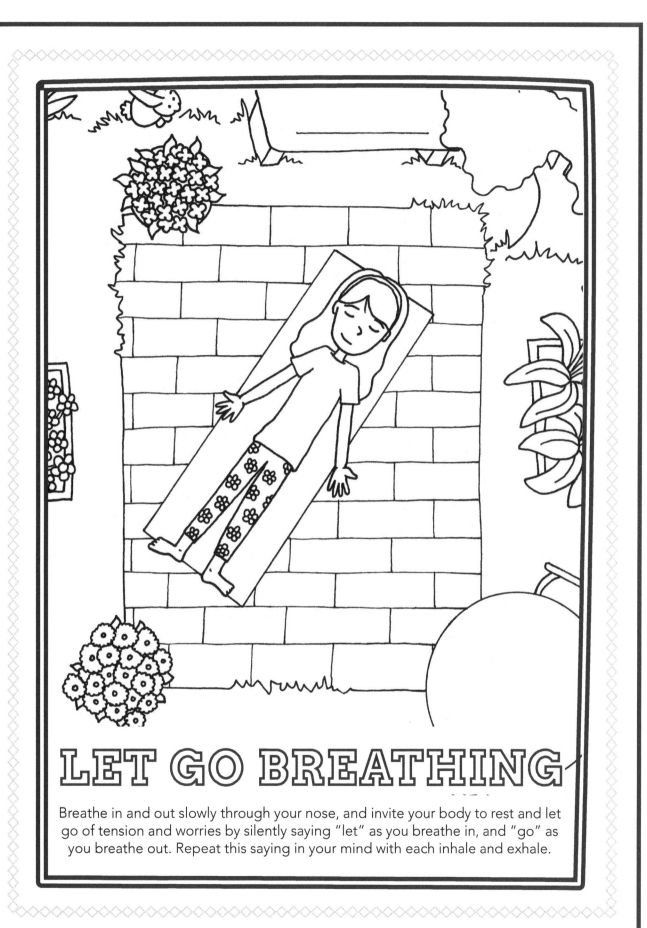

LET GO BREATHING

Breathe in and out slowly through your nose, and invite your body to rest and let go of tension and worries by silently saying "let" as you breathe in, and "go" as you breathe out. Repeat this saying in your mind with each inhale and exhale.

Use This Space to Draw
Your Own Poses or Activities

Can you create something brand new?

Use This Space to Draw Your Own Poses or Activities

Can you create something brand new?

Use This Space to Draw Your Own Poses or Activities

Can you create something brand new?

Use This Space to Draw Your Own Poses or Activities

Can you create something brand new?